A Concise Introduction To Indian Medicine

INDIAN MEDICAL TRADITION

Edited by

DOMINIK WUJASTYK

&

KENNETH G. ZYSK

Vol. VIII

A Concise Introduction to Indian Medicine

(La Médecine indienne)

GUY MAZARS

Translated by
T. K. GOPALAN

MOTILAL BANARSIDASS PUBLISHERS
PRIVATE LIMITED • DELHI

First Editon : Delhi, 2006

ISBN: 81-208-3058-X

MOTILAL BANARSIDASS
41 U.A. Bungalow Road, Jawahar Nagar, Delhi 110 007
8 Mahalaxmi Chamber, 22 Bhulabhai Desai Road, Mumbai 400 026
203 Royapettah High Road, Mylapore, Chennai 600 004
236, 9th Main III Block, Jayanagar, Bangalore 560 011
Sanas Plaza, 1302 Baji Rao Road, Pune 411 002
8 Camac Street, Kolkata 700 017
Ashok Rajpath, Patna 800 004
Chowk, Varanasi 221 001

PRINTED IN INDIA
BYJAINENDRA PRAKASH JAIN AT SHRI JAINENDRA PRESS,
A-45 NARAINA, PHASE-I, NEW DELHI 110 028
AND PUBLISHED BYNARENDRA PRAKASH JAIN FOR
MOTILAL BANARSIDASS PUBLISHERS PRIVATE LIMITED,
BUNGALOW ROAD, DELHI 110 007

CONTENTS

FOREWORD

Guy Mazars' introduction to traditional Indian medicine has been available to the French-reading public for ten years.[1] It is a small masterpiece of clarity, presenting in a few pages a great deal of accurate and historically-informed information about the healing traditions of India, and especially Āyurveda.

During the twentieth century, much debate took place concerning the appropriate way to modernize Āyurveda within India.[2] How could Āyurveda be practised most appropriately in modern India, what should be its relationship with modern establishment medicine? In more recent decades, Āyurveda has been going through the further process of globalization. Clinics from Madras to Manhattan now offer therapies in the name of Āyurveda. Many international cosmetic and health retail chains offer products branded as āyurvedic.[3] The term 'New Age Āyurveda' has been coined to describe these new forms that the tradition is taking.[4] In spite of the fact that 'authenticity' is watchword for these commodified forms of Āyurveda, almost none of these products or therapies would have been recognised by an āyurvedic physician practising in India even two hundred years ago. The changes implicit in modernization are inevitable, and need not to be condemned, but to be understood.

The need for trustworthy information is a critical issue for Āyurveda. It is difficult for either doctors or patients to lay hands on genuinely reliable information about the background and meaning of āyurvedic medicine. And as governments outside India start to require the establishment of regulatory bodies and professional associations, the need for sound information becomes critical, if modernized Āyurveda is not to be branded as quack medicine. The last decade has seen an explosion in the publication of popular works promoting Āyurveda as a new therapy for the West, as well as for the westernized middle classes in India. All these books are written by authors who are primarily interested in promoting Āyurvedic therapy in practice. Almost none of these authors has either a critical awareness of historical issues bearing on Āyurveda, or any linguistic ability in Sanskrit, the language in which all the classic works on Āyurveda up to the nineteenth century are written. On the other hand, they often have a strong vested interest in increasing their client base or promoting product sales. The dominance of this kind of literature is not useful when trying to come to a balanced and properly informed opinion about āyurvedic medicine. But it often seems to be the only literature easily available through normal channels. There is a strong need for informational works which are based on scholarly University-level research, such as the one presented here.

Guy Mazars' book is based on the first-hand study of the original Sanskrit literature of Āyurveda as well as a life-long engagement with ethnobotany, and the observation of ayurvedic practice in contemporary India. It is a great pleasure now to be able to present a new English translation, specially commissioned for the series *Indian Medical Tradition.*

—Dominik Wujastyk
Kenneth G. Zysk

---

1. G. Mazars. *La médecine indienne.* Que Sais-je? Presses Universitaires de France, Paris, 1995.
2. D. Wujastyk. 'Policy formation and debate concerning the government regulation of ayurveda in Great Britain in the 21st century.' *Asian Medicine: Tradition and Modernity,* 1:162-84,2005.
3. E Zimmermann. 'Gentle purge: the flower power of āyurveda.' In C. Leslie and A. Young, editors, *Paths to Asian Medical Knowledge,* pages 209-223. University of California Press, Berkeley, Oxford, etc., 1992.
4. K. G. Zysk. 'New Age Āyurveda or what happens to Indian mediicne when it comes to America.' *Traditional South Asian Medicine,* 6:10-26, 2001

NOTE ON THE TRANSCRIPTION

a is pronounced as **u** in *but*

i is pronounced as **i** in *bit*

u is pronounced as **u** in *put*

ā, ī, ū are longer forms of **a, i, u** above

e and **o** are always long

ṛ is pronounced approximately as **ri**

c is pronounced as **ch** in *chin*

g is pronounced as **g** in *gun*

ṭ, ḍ, ṇ are pronounced with retroflexion of the tip of the tongue towards the back of the palate

s is always as in *say*

ś as **ch** in the German word *ich*

ṣ as **sh** in *shore*

ṃ is called *anusvāra,* and nasalises the preceding vowel.

Introduction

The coexistence of western medicine and so-called 'traditional' systems of medicine is a feature of all health systems outside Europe. In Asia, traditional systems of medicine often cover more than 80 per cent of health requirements. India, the land of spices and the cradle of Yoga, is also one of the regions of the world where, far from disappearing in the face of the success of modern medicine introduced by Europeans, these systems of medicine are still widely practised and offer advantages that meet the concerns of the World Health Organization. There are scholarly forms of these systems, inherited from ancient medical systems, based on written traditions, and popular forms transmitted orally. All of them evoke a growing interest among Western anthropologists, physicians and pharmacologists.

The most widespread of these systems, and the most famous, is Āyurveda, the Science (*veda*) of longevity (*āyur*), an ancient medical system whose main theories were already fixed more than two thousand years ago. As we know from the oldest texts which have come down to us, Āyurveda is first and foremost remarkable for its scientific purpose. It may be described as based on reasoned observation, and offers a rudimentary but rational system of interpretation of the constitution of the body, its vital functions and diseases, according to a holistic approach to man that includes all somatic and psychic symptoms.

In the Western world, Āyurveda was unknown for a very long time outside a few specialist circles. It is only during the last ten or fifteen years that some āyurvedic practices (or what are so described) have begun to spread in America and Europe, especially in Germany, Italy and France. Unfortunately, this popularisation has not always been accompanied, until now, by a critical reflection on the authenticity, safety and efficacy of practices whose antiquity and efficacy tend, too often to be exaggerated by the western press.

In this little book, I have endeavoured to present an overall view of the traditional medicine of India from its origins until the present day, describing in turn its history, its theoretical foundations, its methods of prevention and treatment, the medical profession and lastly its present status and future prospects.

CHAPTER 1

INDIAN MEDICINE ACROSS THE CENTURIES

The earliest data concerning the science and practice of medicine in India come to us from the material remains of the so-called "Indus valley" civilisation (2500-1500 BC). But it is mostly from the sacred texts of the *vedic* religion that one can gain an idea of the medical art in India up to the advent of Buddhism. The concepts that were developed during the *vedic* period were to serve as the basis of a scholarly medicine which has had immense success in the entire Indian world and even beyond.

I. From the Origins to the Birth of Āyurveda

The remains of Mohenjo-Daro in the lower Indus valley and of Harappā, further north, attest to the existence of a civilisation of such a high level, from as early as the third millennium BC, that we may safely think that medicine might have already been very advanced there, but they do not tell us anything as regards its actual development. We know that these cities had trade relations with Mesopotamia, as proved by the discoveries at Ur, Susa or Kish, in strata of the third millennium BC, of seals and other objects coming manifestly from the Indus. These commercial relations perhaps favoured the exchange, if not of scientific concepts or theories, at least of practical knowledge and of medical formulas, between the two civilisations. Now, since this epoch, there were already physicians in Mesopotamia who possessed a considerable knowledge of the curative powers of a number of plants and remedies of mineral and animal origin.[1]

Certain substances discovered in the ruins of Mohenjo-Daro or Harappā may have served as remedies. Thus, the horns of a member of the cervidae family, the *sambar*, evidently preserved for their own sake since they have been discovered without any other remains of the animal, may have had a therapeutic use. Reduced to powder, they are still used in popular Indian medicine. Bones of cuttlefish and bitumen have also been found and they have long figured in Āyurvedic pharmacopoeia. Unfortunately, the use of such substances proves nothing as regards the medical knowledge of those who were using them.

Excavations have above all revealed installations of public and private baths, connected by terracotta pipes to a system of main sewers which follow the layout of the streets. At Mohenjo-Daro, the largest edifice comprises a 13m by 7m tank, with vast outbuildings. These remarkable structures, without parallel in antiquity, are evidence of a concern for hygiene which, while not necessarily being founded on conceptions of prophylaxis and therapeutics, constituted a response to the insalubriousness of the Indus valley.

In the absence of supplementary evidence, it has not been possible to determine the magnitude of the medical legacy from which the Aryan immigrants may have benefited. In any case these immigrants possessed, when they arrived, in the course of the second millennium BC, if not an elaborate medical doctrine,[2] at least a certain number of notions which later contributed to the formation of a physiology and a cosmology. They concern notably the cosmic and somatic role of water, fire and air, and appear in the oldest layer of vedic literature, that of the *Saṃhitā*s or "collections" of hymns, liturgical chants and sacrificial or magical formulas, which constitute the *Veda* proper (1500-1000 BC). The numerous allusions in the vedic *Saṃhitās* to the parts of the body, to the organs and to the diseases and their treatment are complemented by the information in the *Brāhmaṇa*s and older *Upaniṣad*s, which correspond to the period of about 1000 to 500 before the beginning of the Christian era. In the absence of a descriptive text, the information that we can glean from them enables us to have an idea of the rudiments one might have possessed in that epoch concerning anatomy, physiology, diseases and therapeutics.

A number of parts of the body are given a special name or several names in the *Saṃhitās*. They are found especially in magical invocations in which the different parts of the body are named for exorcising the ailments which have established themselves in them, or else in the passages which establish a parallel between the constituents of the body and those of the universe. They are not restricted to the human body, but include animal body parts as well. Some are concerned also with the organs of animals such as the cow or the goat dismembered during sacrifices (*Atharvaveda*, IX, 5; X, 9-10). In all, the anatomical nomenclature of the *Saṃhitās* comprises more than 300 terms. In addition to those which denote the visible parts of the body, there are some which relate to internal organs, but the notions covered by them are fairly rudimentary. Furthermore, many of these terms are metaphorical or periphrastic designations which have not been sanctioned by the usage of language. By contrast, several of the names of organs or organic constituents attested in the Saṃhitās have passed into classical Sanskrit and figure in the medical texts. Thus, the *Saṃhitās* mention the principal constituents of the body, already in part as they were to be known later in classical medicine. Several, like the blood (*rakta*), the flesh (*māṃsa*), the bones (*asthi*) or the fat (*medas*), are the result of common observation. Others, like the *rasa*, or the *ojas*, correspond rather to theoretical conceptions which were to remain in vogue in classical medical doctrine. In the *Ṛgveda* the word *rasa* denotes an organic "juice" which plays an important role in fertilisation. As regards *ojas*, which is described by later medical texts as a substance whose presence in the body is necessary for life, it is no doubt scarcely different from the *ojas* which in the *Saṃhitās* constitutes the strength of the god Indra. The *Saṃhitās* mention also another organic fluid, the bile *(pitta)* which already appears as an element related to fire.

The ideas which vedic authors might have had about the functioning of the organism are connected with their conception of air as the soul of the world, the force which animates the Macrocosm as well as the Microcosm. The whole of physiology rests on the circulation of organic "breaths". An examination of the principal *Saṃhitās* which contain the names of these breaths shows that, from the time of their redaction, pneumatic physiology, which later dominated Indian medicine and yoga, was already in the process of formation. Five breaths are frequently mentioned in the *Saṃhitās*, mainly in Book X of the *Ṛgveda* and in Book XV of the *Atharvaveda*.

The *Saṃhitās* make allusion to a great number of diseases. Their names appear especially in the formulas of the *Atharvaveda* intended to combat them. But, for want of a systematic description of these morbid states, their identification remains uncertain and generally imprecise. One of the diseases whose name occurs most often in the texts is *yakṣma* which is found especially associated with affections leading to a wasting away that is either general or limited to certain parts of the body. The *Atharvaveda* informs us fairly well about fevers, which it denotes by the name of *takman* and of which it lists all the recognised types. Most of the other affections mentioned are most often symptomatic accidents which were then considered as so many separate morbid entities. This is the case with cough or headaches. A "backache" applies no doubt to lumbago. A word which means "lance", *suśūla*, denotes shooting pain, especially in the expression *karṇaśūla*, "earache". The "flow", *āsrāva*, must certainly mean all kinds of excessive flow resulting from urinary or digestive affections. Finally, terms that are ordinarily translated by "leprosy" and "scabies" can denote all sorts of skin lesions, for nothing proves that the clinical entities to which we have given these names were already clearly individualised diseases during the *vedic* epoch. Some indications can nevertheless lead us to think that there was a progress towards the conception of single morbid entities with multiple symptoms. Thus, fever is declared to be the "sister" or "cousin" of other symptoms.

However the true cause of various diseases was not known. Their origins, when they are reported, are in the realm of magic rather than in that of pathogenesis. Indeed, most of the affections named are generally considered as the consequence of an infringement of *ṛta*, that is to say the cosmic as well as moral order of the world, and described as the work of offended deities or evildoing entities, demons and magicians. This notion of *ṛta*, according to which everything is governed by a regular universal law, goes back to the Indo–Iranian period. Founded on the observation of the regularity of natural phenomena, like the alternation of days and nights and the return of the seasons, it was extended to living beings whose behaviour it was supposed to regulate. In relation to such a conception, every infringement, voluntary or not, of the moral code appears as a transgression of *ṛta*, which manifests as a disorder in the organism. Disease is thus closely connected with sin. Dropsy is considered, for example, as the punishment by the god Varuṇa, the guardian of *ṛta*.

Vedic therapeutics is mostly magical. It starts with the principle that gods can suspend the automatic mechanism of retribution for the faults committed. Therapeutics is constituted mostly by formulas which must be recited to implore the pardon of the gods, expel the demons or break the spells of sorcerers. Their recitation was accompanied by magical operations having the purpose of strengthening the efficacy of the curative charms which consisted most often in rituals of cleansing destined to erase the fault that is at the origin of the disease. These rituals have been preserved for us in the texts attached to the *Atharvaveda*, like the *Kauśikasūtra* and in works of the same nature. However, the effects of some plants on the organism did not go unnoticed, and their use for therapeutic purposes is attested from the vedic period, as testified by a well-known hymn of the *Atharvaveda* which is devoted to them. But most of them must have played more often the role of magical ingredients than that of true drugs. It is notably the case of a gum resin which was administered orally to obtain the healing of wounds, in the evident hope that it would close them up, like it closes up the notches of the trees, out of which it oozes. The behaviour of sick animals was also noticed. We read for example in the *Atharvaveda* (VIII, 7, 23): "The wild boar knows the plant which cures, and the mongoose also knows it." This example reminds us that of the shepherd Melampus who, according to Theophrastus (327-287 BC), discovered the purgative properties of hellebore by seeing the effect which it had on his sheep. Such allusions testify in addition to the role played by observation in the discovery and selection of medicinal plants.

It was only towards the end of the vedic period that Indian medicine began to become observational and rational and progressively constitute itself into a consistent system to which the name of Āyurveda, the "Science (*veda*) concerning longevity (*āyur*)", was given. The legends related by the ancient Sanskrit medical texts make of this system a revealed "science", annexed to the *Veda* sometimes as an "annexed member" (*upāṅga*) of the *Atharvaveda*, sometimes as a "sub-veda" (*upaveda*) of the *Ṛgveda*. Created by Brahman and transmitted to men by the successive interventions of Prajāpati, the *Aśvins* and Indra, this science is theoretically divided into eight branches:

i. General surgery;
ii. Oto-rhino-laryngology and ophthalmology;
iii. General therapeutics;
iv. Toxicology;
v. Demonology;
vi. Obstetrics and pediatrics;
vii. Tonic medicine;
viii. Aphrodisiac medicine.

In fact, very few ancient texts follow this division which has been particularly in vogue among more recent authors. As regards their content, it represents in reality the fruit of the activity of medical observation and speculation in the course of the seven or eight centuries which preceded the Christian era. Unfortunately the documents going back to this period that are properly medical have disappeared, and they have been supplanted by more recent texts. Allusions found in a certain number of Sanskrit texts and the testimonies left for us by the Greeks who were contemporaries of Alexander the Great nevertheless enable us to have an idea of some of the progress achieved in relation to the medicine of the vedic era. Thus, Buddhist texts mention already in the entourage of Buddha (sixth or fifth century BC) a celebrated physician by the name of Jīvaka, to whom tradition attributes extraordinary operations, such as laparotomies and skull trepanning, which are reported to have been made under anaesthesia with Indian hemp. Secondly it has been recognised by general agreement that the theory of Āyurvedic physiopathology must have been entirely constituted at the time of the grammarian Kātyāyana (fourth century BC). Onesicrates reports at about the same period that Indians owed their longevity to a perfect hygiene and that the Gymnosophists were doing great research on natural phenomena and diseases. Megasthenes, who lived for a long time in India as ambassador, at a period close to 300 BC, gives us more precise indications which agree fully with the Indian data. In particular, his testimony regarding the treatment given to elephants shows that in this area veterinary medicine was already what we learn from later texts on elephantology. A certain amount of data concerning medicines and therapeutics are provided to us by the *Arthaśāstra*, a treatise on statecraft attributed to Kauṭilya, *alias* Cāṇakya, minister of Candragupta (313-289 BC), the founder of the Mauryan dynasty in India. They already suppose the existence of a medical doctrine fairly close to that which is revealed to us by the treatises of Āyurveda.

II. The Period of the Great Medical Corpuses

The classic doctrine of Āyurveda is already found fully developed in two voluminous treatises dating from the beginning of the Christian era, the *Carakasaṃhitā* (Caraka's collection) and the *Suśrutasaṃhitā* (Susruta's collection), which are the oldest Sanskrit medical texts that have come down to us. Although these two works agree remarkably in their general teachings, they are too different for us to suppose that one may be the imitation of the other. But they manifestly rely on the same older doctrinal heritage.

The *Carakasaṃhitā* is supposed to contain the teachings of the sage Ātreya Punarvasu, recorded by one of his disciples, Agniveśa, and revised by Caraka. Ātreya and Agniveśa belong to the realm of legend, but Caraka is likely to have been a historical figure. Indeed, according to Buddhist sources, a physician of the same name was practising at the court of the Indo-Scythian king Kaniṣka (first and second centuries AD). Like Aśoka (264-227 BC) some centuries earlier, Kaniṣka was well-disposed towards Buddhism and protected it. During his reign, Indian, Sanskritic and Buddhist cultures hold a great expansion. The redaction of the *Carakasaṃhitā* thus goes back to this period, if it is indeed the same Caraka, which is probable but not certain. However, the text which has come down to us contains more recent portions added at the time of its revision in the ninth century, by an author from Kashmir, Dṛḍhabala. But the core of its content is much older since Caraka himself had only reconstructed an already existing work, cited under the name of *Agniveśatantra*, the "Book of Agniveśa".

The *Suśrutasaṃhitā*, which constitutes the major source of information about Indian surgery, is supposed to contain the teachings of the god Dhanvantari, who was incarnated as Divodāsa, king of Varanasi. Therefore it is not the personal work of Suśruta, who too has only transmitted an already constituted medical tradition. The date of its redaction is not known. The basic text is supposed to have been revised and enlarged by an author called Nāgārjuna whom tradition identifies with the Buddhist philosopher of that name (first and second centuries AD). But it is also possible that the attribution of the name of Nāgārjuna to the reviser of the text is but an echo of the legend which would have the great Buddhist philosopher to be a physician and an alchemist. In any case, the teaching of Suśruta must already have been fixed at the time of the *Carakasaṃhitā* which refers moreover to the disciples of Suśruta for surgical treatment.

Composed without a preestablished didactic plan and principally reflecting oral teachings given from day to day, these two texts were the object, from a period even earlier than the tenth century, of very elaborate commentaries whose purpose was to clarify and add precision to their contents. The *Carakasaṃhitā* was commented upon in the ninth century by Jejjaṭa, then, in the eleventh century, by Cakrapāṇidatta, himself the author of a manual of therapeutics and a treatise of materia medica, both highly valued. The principal commentaries are those of Jejjaṭa, Gayadāsa (XI century) and especially that of Ḍalhaṇa (XI-XII centuries) entitled *Nibandhasaṃgraha.*

Among the other texts which emerged during the classical period, the major ones are the *Bhelasaṃhitā*, the *Aṣṭāṅgasaṃgraha* and the *Aṣṭāṅgahṛdayasaṃhitā*. The *Bhelasaṃhitā*, which is derived from the teachings of Atreya, like the *Carakasaṃhitā*, constitutes a collection quite distinct from *Carakasaṃhitā* and is probably of an earlier date. The *Aṣṭāṅgasaṃgraha* and the *Aṣṭāṅgahṛdayasaṃhitā* are by Vāgbhaṭa, the most celebrated author after Caraka and Suśruta. They are probably two different recensions of the same medical text whose teachings agree generally with those of Caraka and Suśruta. But the more commonly used text of Vāgbhaṭa is the *Aṣṭāṅgahṛdayasaṃhitā*. It is not known at what period Vāgbhaṭa lived. It seems that he must be placed in the sixth century or a little after it. He is in any case earlier than the tenth century. His identity has been the subject of unending discussion, and Indian critics hold that there was an "elder Vāgbhaṭa" in addition to Vāgbhaṭa, grandson of the former and son of Siṃhagupta. The Chinese pilgrim Y Jing, who visited India from 673 to 695, spoke, without mentioning its name, of a work that was then recent and that summarised the eight branches of medicine. It is thought that he was referring to the work of Vāgbhaṭa, but he may also have been referring to the *Yogaśataka*, "The Hundred Formulas of Yoga", which fits Yi Jing's description perfectly. This summarised form of medicine consists, as its name indicates, of a series of one hundred therapeutic formulas distributed according to the eight theoretical divisions of Āyurveda. Its author is a certain Nāgārjuna, perhaps the same author who is reputed to have revised the *Suśrutasaṃhitā* but who is not necessarily the Buddhist patriarch of that name with whom he is nevertheless identified by tradition. To a Nāgārjuna is also attributed a manual on sorcery, the *Kakṣapuṭa*, and a text on alchemy, the *Rasendramaṅgala*. The alchemist Nāgārjuna, who is mentioned by Somadeva (eleventh century) in his *Kathāsaritsāgara* and by the Jaina monk Merutuṅga (twelfth century) in his *Prabandhacintāmaṇi*, is reputed to have lived in the tenth century.

Alongside the great classical treatises and their commentaries there exists an abundant medical literature that comprises other general texts, specialised manuals and repertories of materia medica. Mādhavakara, an author of the eighth century, has left a *Rogaviniścaya*, "Diagnosis of Diseases", better known under the title of "*Mādhavanidāna*", "Etiology according to Mādhava", in which he treats specially causes and symptoms of the different diseases, by taking up in a systematic manner the data of Caraka, Suśruta and Vāgbhaṭa. It is probably around the year 1000 that Vṛnda wrote his *Siddhayoga*, "Perfect Preparations" which follows the treatise of Mādhavakara step-by-step, complementing it with a mass of data relating to therapeutics. A collection of therapeutics of the same kind was written by Vaṅgasena (probably between 1050 and 1100).

III. The Development of Āyurveda

Once they had been fixed, the āyurvedic doctrines of interpretation of the constitution of the body, the vital functions and the diseases scarcely varied in the course of the centuries that followed, probably for want of acquisition of new knowledge concerning anatomy and physiology. It must be said that a very severe blow was administered by the Muslim invasions to the thirst for discovery and to the ancient spirit of scientific research in India. In the face of foreign doctrines that arrived in India, the āyurvedic circles thought more of asserting the value of their system in its established form than facilitating its development by new research. By contrast, a large number of acquisitions by way of details took place in the area of diagnostic methods and especially in the area of therapeutics.

One of the major innovations is the examination of the pulse (*nāḍīparīkṣā*) which does not seem to be known before the eighth century. The treatises of Caraka, Suśruta and Vāgbhaṭa do not speak of it. The method was described only in the *Śārṅgadharasaṃhitā* (thirteenth or fourteenth century) and a certain number of small texts of uncertain date but that are manifestly more recent and entirely devoted to it, like the *Nāḍīvijñāna* attributed to Kaṇāda. It was thought that the idea might have been borrowed from China but the Indian method is different.

There are also divergencies between the nosology described in the *Śārṅgadharasaṃhitā* and the nosological system of the *Mādhavanidāna*. New names of diseases are mentioned in the texts. Syphilis is described for the first time, under the name of *phiraṅgaroga*, in the *Bhāvaprakāśa* of Bhāvamiśra (sixteenth century).

After the period of the great medical texts, new drugs, like opium, were introduced into the pharmacopoeia, while plants already known were promoted to the rank of panaceas. It is especially the case with *harītakī* (chebulic myrobalan), Terminalia Chebula Retz, which Caraka classifies under the name of *abhayā* among the plants against hemorrhoids and skin diseases. Foreign substances made their appearance in food prescriptions, like the chilli, of South American origin and introduced by the Portuguese. We notice moreover the appearance of a larger number of mineral preparations whose introduction into therapeutics coincided with the development of alchemy during the medieval period. Alchemical texts give us a large number of recipes for elixirs (*rasāyana*), unguents (*pralepa*) and pills (*guṭikā*) intended to preserve the body from old age and even from death. They are often preparations made from mercury salts (*pārada*) which are believed to confer, besides immortality and youthfulness, all kinds of extraordinary powers or *siddhis*, like that of flying through the air or transmuting base metals into silver or gold. Alchemic therapy occupies a very important place in Siddha medicine.

IV. Siddha Medicine and Greco–Arab Medicine

Alongside Āyurveda a fairly rich iatrochemistry was formed, with several traditions one of which is represented by what is known as Siddha medicine. The Siddhas or "Perfect Ones" are yogis, iatrochemists and alchemists, very often legendary figures, who owe especially their name to the *siddhis* or "perfections", the terms denoting the extraordinary powers which are attributed to them, such as the transmission of thought, action from afar on objects, clairvoyance, invisibility, levitation and the power of transmuting metals.

Several movements, in the course of the Middle Ages, claimed to derive their inspiration from these Siddhas. Among these movements, there is one which has adherents even today, that of the Nātha-yogin which derives its name from the title of *nātha*, "protector", reserved to its spiritual masters. One of them, Gorakṣanātha, is reputed to have popularised the techniques of haṭhayoga across the entire Indian continent. The tradition of this movement recognises nine *Nāthas* and 84 *Siddhas*. Sanskrit literature has preserved only some traces of their activities. But the legendary accounts of their lives, and their teachings, have been preserved for us by the Tibetan tradition.

Today, this medicine is especially practised in Tamilnadu, in the south of India, where the literature of this school is reputed to have been elaborated by a group of 18 *Cittar* (Tamil form of the Sanskrit *Siddha*). Many texts have been published since the middle of the last century but, in the absence of any chronology, it is difficult to fix with any certainty the period of their redaction. Several of these texts are attributed to Akattiyar (Agastya of the Sanskrit texts), the legendary civiliser of the Tamil country.[3]

Some admirers of Siddha medicine do not hesitate to push its origins back to a period much earlier than that of the arrival of the Aryans in India. Conversely, many specialists of Āyurveda recognise no originality in Siddha medicine.

Founded in fact on the same general principles as Āyurveda, from which it is manifestly derived in part, Siddha medicine also shows original aspects which were able in their turn to influence, to a certain extent, the development of Āyurveda during the medieval period.

In particular, the teachings of Siddha medicine rely on special anatomical and physiological conceptions which have also played an important role in the development of haṭhayoga and tantrism.

Siddha medicine also distinguishes itself from Āyurveda by the place occupied by the examination of the pulse in the determination of the diagnosis. There are several well-known Tamil works concerning the pulse and the blood vessels, like the *Kurunāṭicāstiram* or "Treatise on the kuru vessels" attributed to the Cittar Akattiyar. These works distinguish several kinds of pulses, according to the strength and the rhythm of the pulsations. These pulsations are considered as the reflection of the activity of a central vital current, the *kurunāṭi*, showing the variations in the functioning of vital principles. Finally, the therapeutics is characterised by a great number of remedies based on mineral and acid products, and various salts.

Greco–Arab medicine was introduced into the Indian subcontinent as a result of the Muslim invasions, and became established there from the twelfth century. It continued to develop there, long after its decline in the West, mostly among the Muslim population. It has retained an honourable place there under the name of unānī medicine,[4] a name which originally meant "Greek", or more exactly "Ionian" (Sanskrit *yavana*).

Arabic medicine, let us remember, is neither Muslim nor the exclusive work of the Arabs. It is only the language of this medicine that is Arabic, and this language had been the vehicle of science between the nations of Europe and Asia from the ninth to the fourteenth century. This medicine took shape in the course of the first two centuries after the Hejira from the old medical knowledge of the Sumerians, the Babylonians and the Assyrians, to which was added that of the Greeks, with in addition the borrowings from Iran and even from India.

Under the reign of Alā'ud-Dīn Khalji (1296-1316), there were a number of *hakīms* (the name given to the Arabian physicians) at Delhi and also famous practitioners of Āyurveda, if we are to believe the testimony of the historian Baranī (fourteenth century). Under the reign of Muḥammad ben Tughluq, sultan from 1325 to 1351, there were 70 dispensaries and hospitals in Delhi alone employing a large number of doctors. It was at the demand of this monarch that Hakīm Ḍiyā Muḥammad, son of Muḥammad Mas'ūd, wrote (around 1336) his *Majmū-e Ḍiyā'ī*, in which a whole chapter is devoted to the "medicine of Nāgārjuna and the other yogis of India". From this period dates also the *Kitāb al-Kulliyāt wa Juziyāt* of Ḍiyā al-Dīn Bakhshi on Indian medicinal plants (herbs and bushes). Fīrūz Shāh Tughluq, the successor of Muḥammad ben Tughluq was himself a physician and, it would appear, an excellent bonesetter. He was especially interested in ophthalmology. There is a collyrium whose composition is attributed to him and which moreover bears his name. It is under his rule and according to his instructions that the *Ṭibb-e-Fīrūz* was compiled. Some years later Shihab al-Dīn Abd'al-Karim Nagori wrote a treatise of therapeutics, the *Ṭibb-e-Shihabi.*

Following the example of the sultans of Delhi, many Muslim princes of India encouraged medicine. Thus, under the reign of Maḥmūd Shāh of Gujarat (between 1458 and 1511) several texts on āyurvedic medicine were translated including the *Aṣṭāṅgahṛdayasaṃhitā* of Vāgbhaṭa under the title *Ṭibb-e-Shifā-e-Maḥmūd-Shāhī.* Another important work is the *Ma'dan al-Shifā' Sikandar Shāhī* of Mian Bhowa *alias* Bahwa bin Khawās Khān (1512) which is a compilation of āyurvedic medical texts, done under the reign of Sikandar Shāh Lodī (1489-1517).

The golden age of unani medicine was during the period of the Great Mughals (sixteenth to seventeenth centuries) when several Hakīms were attracted to their court. India then became the refuge of Arabic medicine whose most active centres were Lahore, Delhi, Lucknow, Patna, Murshidabad, Hyderabad and Madras. Among the most important authors of this period we must mention Hakīm 'Ali Gīlānī, an Iranian physician and mathematician hailing from Gīlān (in Iran), who arrived in India under the reign of Akbar (1556-1605). We owe to him especially the *Sharh-e Qānūn-e ibn Sīnā*, in Arabic, which is a commentary on the *Canon* of Avicenna (in 1613). Subsequently unani medicine continued to develop during the reigns of Jahāngīr (1605-1627) and Shāhjahān (1627-1657) and culminated under the reign of Aurangzeb (1657-1707).

The foundations of this unani medicine are those of Arabic medicine, themselves inherited from the Greek medical science. The technical terms are moreover mostly Arabic, the Arabic words being often nothing more than simple transliterations of the Greek. But one encounters also several notions unknown to Greek medicine and to the earlier texts of Arabic medicine, notably in the area of physiology. As regards therapeutics, it must have been adapted to the geographical and climatic conditions of the Indian subcontinent, taking largely into account the acquisitions of āyurvedic medicine.

V. The Spread of Āyurveda

Āyurveda has had a vast area of expansion. Much before the expedition of Alexander the Great, communications between Greece and India were easy through the Achemenid empire of Persia. One could travel from India to Greece not only by reaching Ionia from the south or from the centre of Asia Minor, but also by the Pontus Euxinus and Thrace. There was no dearth of intermediaries, such as the Greeks who were at the service of the Achemenids who ruled at the same time over Greek and Indian lands, and Indians themselves, for facilitating scientific exchanges between India and Greece, in parallel with commercial relations. If Aristoxenus of Tarantum is to be believed, as quoted, from Aristocles, by Eusebius in his *Praeparatio Evangelica* (XI, 3, 8), an Indian sage even met Socrates at Athens. It is known moreover that Egyptian, Greek and Indian physicians competed with each other at the court of Susa. Dioscorides and Pliny described a number of Indian drugs.

Later on, Indian medicine was taught in Susiana, at the school of Jundishapur founded in the fifth century by the Nestorians.[5] It must probably have been due to the fame that it had acquired in Persia before Islamisation that it was actively studied at the beginning of the formation of Arabic medicine.[6] Indeed, a Persian version of *Carakasaṃhitā* had been translated into Arabic by the time of the first 'Abbasīd khalifs (eighth century), as testified by the *Kitāb al-Fihrist* of Ibn an-Nadīm, completed according to the assertion of its author himself in 998 of the Christian era. Under the reign of the famous Khalifa Hārūn al-Rashīd (786-809), the treatise of Suśruta (*Susrud* in Arabic) was translated, as well as other works. Hārūn al-Rashīd himself is believed to have been treated by an Indian physician. Arab texts cite the translations of *Mādhavanidāna* and *Aṣṭāṅgahṛdayasaṃhitā*. A very complete summary of the āyurvedic doctrines is given to us in the *Firdaws al-Ḥikmat* written in 850 by 'Alī Ibn Rabban aṭ-Ṭabarī. In the tenth century, the pharmacologist Abū Manṣūr Muwaffaq ibn 'Alī al-Harawī used, alongside Greek sources, a number of materials of Indian origin, to compose his treatise on the properties of the drugs entitled *Kitāb al-abnīya 'an ḥaqā'īq al-adwīya.* Abū Bakr Muḥammad ar-Rāzī, better known under the name of Rhazes, also knew Indian medicine, as proved by his citations of Suśruta. For his part, the biographer Ibn abī Uṣaybi'a (1194-1270) attests that many Indian physicians had been known to Arabs and Persians.

But it is above all in the lands where Indian culture had been introduced with Buddhism that Āyurveda obtained the greatest success. For Buddhism has always attached great importance to physical health and the existence of Buddhist hospitals and dispensaries has played a great role in the propagation of Indian medical theories and therapeutics. Buddhist literature, and in particular the Pali Canon, contains a large number of examples of medical science.[7] There is even a hypothesis that there existed a Buddhist medicine which rekindled Āyurveda. It is true that certain medical texts attributed to Buddhist authors, or who called themselves so, are more advanced than the classical treatises of Caraka and Suśruta, but it is simply because they are more recent and less pledged to tradition.

With Buddhism Āyurveda at first penetrated central Asia. Excavations which have been undertaken there, at the end of the nineteenth century and at the beginning of the twentieth, have yielded many medical works. It is thus that, in the region of Kucha, fragments of the *Yogaśataka* have been discovered. In Turkestan, von Le Coq discovered a fragment of the *Bhelasaṃhitā* probably dating from the ninth century.

From central Asia, the reputation of Indian drugs reached China in the second half of the first century, but without being accompanied there by the āyurvedic doctrines which were probably held in check by the existence of a highly developed Chinese medicine. A collection of prescriptions of Sun Simiao (581-682) mentions medicinal plants of Indian origin. The *Haiyo Bencao* or "Maritime Materia Medica" of Li Xun, written under the reign of Su Zong (756-762), gives an account of the drugs imported from India. In Japan, several Indian medicinal plants have been preserved in the treasure house of Shoso-In which was dedicated to the Great Buddha of Nara, after the death of the emperor Shomu-Tenno, around 748.

Indian Āyurveda was popular in Tibet where, as early as from the eighth century, a number of treatises on āyurvedic medicine were translated from Sanskrit into Tibetan, notably the *Aṣṭāṅgahṛdayasaṃhitā* of Vāgbhaṭa and the *Yogaśataka* of Nāgārjuna. Several collections of materia medica and of alchemical texts were also translated into Tibetan and incorporated into the immense Buddhist Encyclopaedia of the *Tanjur* (pronounced /tan dzyur/). We must also stress the importance of these Tibetan translations which in some cases have preserved for us works whose Sanskrit originals have been lost or of which only some fragments have survived. Āyurveda has given to Tibeto–Mongolian medicine the essentials of its classical theoretical foundations and a great part of its practice.[8]

It was also following Buddhism that Āyurveda penetrated Sri Lanka, at the beginning of the Christian era. The Burmese also adopted Indian medicine whose methods competed with Chinese acupuncture in Siam. In Kampuchea, stelae of foundations of hospitals have been found which attest to the development of medical care under the reign of the Buddhist king Jayavarman VII (1181-1218).[9] Today, the traditional medicine of South-East Asia remains profoundly marked by these influences.

VI. Western Medicine and Indian Medicine

Until the end of the fifteenth century, there had only been intermittent contacts between India and Europe. But by reaching the port of Calicut, in 1498, Vasco da Gama gave the Portuguese the possibility of creating an empire. A second voyage, in 1502, took him to Cochin where he established the first Portuguese trading post. The taking of Goa by Albuquerque in 1510 marked the beginning of the European settlement in India. But the Portuguese were only forerunners. They were followed in turn by the Dutch, the British, the Danes and the French in the seventeenth century. Nevertheless, it was the British who were to deploy the most significant activity, after the creation of the *East India Company* (1600). For their part, the French did not remain inactive. In 1664, Colbert created the *Compagnie des Indes orientales*, and, in 1670, a French squadron commanded by admiral La Haye arrived in the Bay of Bengal and launched an attack on San Thomé (near Madras). Shortly thereafter, in 1673, the French settled down in Pondicherry. However, in the eighteenth century, after the eviction of the French (1740-1763) and the fall of Mysore (1799), the last great independent power of the Deccan, the British rapidly extended their rule over the rest of India.

One of the first European physicians in India was the Portuguese Garcia da Orta. He arrived in Goa in 1534, and remained in India until his death in 1570. In the next century, a Frenchman, François Bernier (1620-1688), a doctor of medicine of the Faculty of Montpellier, practised at Aurangzeb's court. From 1674, a French surgeon was present at San Thomé. But it was the British who were to develop measures to improve sanitary conditions and further the spread of modern medicine in India, by combating epidemics and by creating the first hospitals and the first medical teaching establishments. From 1784, medical officers of the British army appear alongside the physicians and surgeons of the *East India Company*. Since there were not enough physicians for the task, they appealed, very early, for the cooperation of indigenous auxiliaries, most often recruited from among the traditional local physicians, the "native doctors". But, in the nineteenth century, the creation of medical schools was found to be necessary. In 1822, a Native Medical Institution was founded at Calcutta, offering a three-year course dispensed in the Hindustani language. In 1826, a medical teaching course was inaugurated at the Sanskrit College at Calcutta. The same year, a similar experiment was attempted at Bombay. These initiatives had varying fortunes. In 1835, as a replacement for the Native Medical Institution, the first college of medicine was created at Calcutta, to train auxiliary civil and military surgeons. It was there that the first dissections of the human body and the first anatomical demonstrations were conducted before Indian students. Four years later, a 100-bed hospital was attached to the college where, the following year, the courses were reorganised to meet the norms of the Royal College of Surgeons of England and the Worshipful Society of Apothecaries of London. The duration of the course was then extended to five years. In 1850, this college of medicine had already eight chairs: anatomy, chemistry, materia medica, forensic medicine, surgery, general medicine, obstetrics and ophthalmic surgery. It was attached to the University of Calcutta, when the latter was founded in 1857. Finally, in 1892, the diploma of medicine of the University of Calcutta was recognised by the General Medical Council of Great Britain.

At Bombay, the Grant Medical School was established in 1845. It developed from 1851 by the addition of new departments and, in 1854, it was recognised by the Royal College of Surgeons. At Madras, the School of Medicine founded in 1843 became a college eight years later, recognised in its turn by the Royal College of Surgeons of London in 1855. Soon, these three establishments were found to be insufficient to meet the needs, and new schools were created in other cities. We shall mention also the dates of some important establishments: 1911, Indian Council of Medical Research at Delhi; 1916, first college of medicine for women at Delhi; 1932, All India Institute of Hygiene and Public Health at Calcutta; 1934, Medical Council of India. In 1946, on the eve of independence, there were 28 colleges of medicine in India. Thirty years later their number rose to 106. In the same period, the number of doctors, pharmacists and medical auxiliaries increased considerably. Moreover, the Medical Council of India was reconstituted in 1956, and a number of new organisations were created subsequently.

One of the first tasks of European medicine in India was the fight against epidemic diseases: cholera, plague, smallpox. Cholera, a disease of polluted waters, described under the name of *viṣūcikā* by Suśruta, has struck India with regularity during centuries. It was in 1945 that Indian doctors first defeated it. Plague, which at the beginning of the century had caused hundreds of thousands of deaths every year (more than 940,000 in the year 1905 alone), was also fought successfully. It was even believed to have been eradicated for good until the appearance of a new seat of infection at Surat, in Gujarat, in September 1994. As regards smallpox, it seems to have totally disappeared in our days, thanks to anti-smallpox vaccination. In 1964, in Karnataka (Mysore), one of the biggest states of the Indian Union, the vaccination programme had already covered nearly 85 per cent of the population. The fight against parasitical diseases and against tuberculosis has also made rapid progress. But another scourge threatens India: AIDS. In 1994, the Indian Health Organization estimated that 2.8 million Indians were seropositive. For its part, the Indian National Aids Control Organisation has advanced a smaller but equally alarming figure of 1.5 million seropositives. As regards the number of cases of the disease officially declared, it is reported to have doubled between 1992 and 1993. Another figure that is causing concern is the percentage of seropositivity noted in the blood of voluntary donors. It seems to have doubled in three years.

Since 1920, and especially since 1947, the improvement in living conditions and the advances of medicine have had the consequence of lowering the mortality rate whereas the birth rate has always remained high, resulting in the population problem which India is facing. Until the decennial census of 1921, the Indian population grew slowly, with rates of increase much lower than those of the European countries. But there has subsequently been a considerable increase in the population from 251 million at the time of the census of 1951, which had grown to 844 million at the census of 1991, and is now over one billion. From 1956, in order to arrest the population growth, the ruling circles in India have practised a policy of birth control. But this policy, especially owing to its unpopularity, has not yielded the expected results. The census of 1991 showed an increase of more than 23 per cent in the population in the space of ten years, and according to provisional figures of the latest census of 2001 the decennial growth is a little under 19 per cent.

As in many other countries of Asia, traditional medicine has remained widely accepted in India, especially among the populations to which modern medicine is not yet accessible, either because it is too costly, or because it has not spread sufficiently. Indeed, the majority of doctors with modern training are too often concentrated in big cities, neglecting rural areas where their services are urgently needed. Moreover, many Indians remain convinced of the superiority of āyurvedic medicine over western medicine, for which traditional science has long displayed that attitude of reserve and even systematic ignorance which it adopted, some centuries earlier, when faced with the medicine introduced by the Muslim invaders.

VII. The Revival of Traditional Medicines

The revival of Āyurveda has been furthered, from the nineteenth century, by a number of private initiatives which have resulted in the creation of institutions and associations, often patronised by local authorities.[10]

The All India Ayurvedic Congress was founded in 1907. In 1916, Kavirāj J. Bhushaṇ Roy created the first college of Āyurveda with a hospital at Calcutta, and this establishment later became a government college and bears his name today. In 1921, a "Society for the teaching of medical texts", the *Vaidyaśāstrapīṭhapariṣad* was established in the same city. It has been calculated that from 1935 to 1946 this association has been responsible for the hospitalisation of more than 700 patients per year and has made available more than 80,000 outpatient consultations.

A traditional school of medicine, the Govinda Sundarā Āyurveda Vidyālaya, was founded in 1922 by a physician of traditional medicine, Kavirāj Ramachandra Mallick, with the support of Manindra Chandra Nandy, Mahārājā of Kasimbazar. Some ten years later, Kavirāj Ganganath Sen (1877-1945) founded the *Viśvanātha Āyurveda Mahāvidyālaya*, with the object of restoring Āyurveda to its scientific foundations by introducing the study of modern medicine in his teaching programme. But this type of initiative provoked criticism by partisans of a "pure Āyurveda" (*śuddha-Āyurveda*) hostile to the introduction of modern disciplines in the training programmes.

One also sees the emergence of the first state institutions in this period. In 1924-25, the government of Madras founded the Government School of Indian Medicine. Soon thereafter, similar experiments were made in other provinces: the creation of the Bihar Government Āyurveda Vidyālaya at Jagannathpur, of the Muzaffarpur Government Āyurveda Vidyālaya, of a college of Āyurveda and unani medicine at Delhi, etc.

Between 1921 and 1958, commissions were constituted at various intervals to take stock of the state of traditional medicine and to suggest measures for its revival. It is on the basis of their recommendations that the teaching and practice of Āyurveda have been organised. There actually exists in India a great number of schools of traditional medicine with hospitals of application and health centres. The teaching has been modernised. Modern anatomy and physiology are now studied alongside Sanskrit medical classics. In the Āyurvedic health centres and hospitals, diagnosis is based most often on the clinical characteristics given by the treatises of Caraka, Suśruta, Vāgbhaṭa and Mādhava, but common medical analyses such as urine tests are also used today.

NOTES

1. See P. Herrero, *La thérapeutique mésopotamienne*, edited by Marcel Sigrist, with a preface by François Vallat, Paris, Editions Recherche sur les Civilisations (ERC), 1984, p. 140.

2. Following the work of E. Benveniste, some authors consider that there already existed among the Indo-Europeans a true medical doctrine structured on a trifunctional schema, with a medicine of charms, a medicine of the knife, a medicine derived from herbs, corresponding respectively to the three great cosmic and social functions of magico–religious supremacy, supremacy of war, and supremacy of production attested among the Indo-Europeans (see E. Benveniste, La doctrine médicale des Indo-Europeons, *Revue de l'histoire des religions*, CXXX, 1945, pp. 5-12). It is true that comparison of the passages relating to medicine in the vedic and avestan texts enables us to arrive at a certain number of concordances between the Indian and Iranian medical data. In particular, the *Avesta* and the *Veda* distinguish effectively three methods of overcoming disease, which seem to correspond perfectly to an Indo-European classification, as shown by the existence of a similar tradition in ancient Greece. But such a division of medications into three categories reveals nothing about the existence of "doctrinal conceptions already established from the Indo-Iranian period" (cf. J. Filliozat, *La doctrine classique de la médecine indienne?*, p. 33). Other concordances between the Indian and Iranian sources, notably with regard to the names of some diseases, can be explained by something entirely different from a common origin.

3. Guy Mazars, Les textes médicaux tamouls, *Proceedings of the International Workshop on Priorities in the Study of Indian Medicine* held at the State University of Groningen, 23-27 October 1983, Rijksuniversiteit te Groningen, 1984, pp. 121-29.

4. Concerning this system of medicine the reader may consult: M.Z. Siddiqui, The Unani Tibb (Greek medicine) in India, *A Concise History of Science in India*, New Delhi, Indian National Science Academy, 1971, pp. 268-73; R.L. Verma, The Growth of Greco-Arabian Medicine in Medieval India, *Indian Journal of History of Science*, 5, 1970, pp. 347-63; R.L. Verma and N.H. Keswani, Unani Medicine in Medieval India. Its Teachers and Texts, in N.H. Keswani (Ed.), *The Science of Medicine and Physiological Concepts in Ancient and Medieval India*, New Delhi, All-India Institute of Medical Sciences, 1974, pp. 127-42.

5. Some scholars claim that this school never existed at all and is a figment of imagination created by gradual exaggeration over generations of historians (Arab and European).

6. D.V. Subba Reddy, Influence of Indian Medicine on Arabian and Persian Medical Literature, *Indian Journal of the History of Medicine*, 4(2), 1959, pp. 25-34. See also M. Ullmann, *Die Medizin im Islam*, Leiden, E.J. Brill, 1970, pp. 103-07.

7. J. Mitra, *A Critical Approach of āyurvedic material in Buddhist Literature with special reference to Tripitakaẏ*, Varanasi, Jyotiralok Prakashan, 1985.

8. Guy Mazars, Médecines du Tibet et de la Haute-Asie, *Encyclopédie des médecines naturelles, Physiothérapie-Aromathérapie,* Paris, Editions Techniques, 1991, A-5, pp. 1-12.

9. C. Jacques, Les édits des hôpitaux de Jayavarman VII, *Etudes cambodgiennes*, 13, 1968, pp. 14-17.

10. A. Rosu, Le renouveau contemporain de l'Āyurveda, *Wiener Zeitschrift fur die Kunde Sudasiens*, 26, 1982, pp. 59-82.

CHAPTER 2

THE CONCEPTUAL FOUNDATIONS OF INDIAN MEDICINE

For more than twenty centuries traditional Indian medicine has based its practice on representations and theories which are those of an ancient system whose name, Āyurveda, could be translated by "biology". Indeed, it is not only a medicine but a representation of vital phenomena, whether they be normal or pathological. In this "biology" is incorporated a psychology, for there is no opposition in the Indian thought between the somatic phenomena and the psychic phenomena. Hence, Āyurveda encompasses, besides the rules of medical practice, all organic, biological and psychological conditions of life in health and disease.

I. Philosophical Foundations of Āyurveda

The conceptual edifice of Āyurveda rests on ideas which are those of the philosophy of "counting" or *Sāṃkhya*, a system of thought having as its basis the analysis and classification of the constituents (*tattva*) of the material world. It is not known in fact which of the two systems influenced the other. Some authors consider that āyurvedic doctrines are older than *Sāṃkhya* whose basic text is the *Sāṃkhyakārikā* or "Stanzas of *Sāṃkhya*" (fourth century?). However that may be, according to āyurvedic treatises as well as according to *Sāṃkhya*, the human body is composed of the same gross elements (*bhūta*) that constitute the universe: earth (*prithvī*), water (*āp*), fire (*tejas*), air (*vāyu*) and space (*ākāśa*), represented respectively by the solid parts, the liquids, the body heat, the breath, and the emptiness of the hollow organs.

These gross elements originate in five "essences" (*tanmātra*) or "subtle elements" defined by the *Sāṃkhya* texts: "It is said that space originates in the essence of sound, air in the essence of touch, fire in the essence of form, water in the essence of taste, the earth in the essence of smell. Thus from the five essences the five gross elements are born" (Commentary of Gaudapāda to the *Sāṃkhyakārikā* , 22). These *tanmātra*s are themselves productions of the *prakṛti*, the "Primeval Form", or *Pradhāna*, the "Primordial Foundation" existing throughout eternity on an equal footing with a spiritual principle, the *Puruṣa*, "Man", single in its essence but countless in its manifestations. Medical texts are also aware of the conceptions of *Sāṃkhya* relating to the three properties (*guṇa*) of the *prakṛti* which serve to categorise people: purity (*sattva*), passion (*rajas*) and darkness (*tamas*) which correspond to each of the three temperaments recognised by Āyurveda. The combinations of the five gross elements form the differentiated substances of the organism, the *dhātu*, seven in number: chyle (*rasa*), blood (*rakta*), flesh (*māṃsa*), fat (*medas*), bone (*asthi*), marrow (*majjā*) and semen (*śukra*).

As it is described in the great treatises of Caraka and Suśruta, āyurvedic medicine distinguishes itself explicitly from empiricism, magic and religion. For, the conditions for the validity of the observations and reasoning which are at the root of diagnosis, prognosis and treatment interested the āyurvedic circles very early. Thus, the *Carakasaṃhitā* contains a teaching of logic intended to guide the future physician in his reasoning. Long passages and allusions appearing in various parts of the treatise constitute the exposition of this logic. The most systematic passages are found in chapters IV and VIII of the section of the *Carakasaṃhitā* entitled Vimānasthāna. Cakrapāṇidatta wrote a detailed commentary on it in the eleventh century, which testifies to the continuity of the scientific tradition. This logic, allied to the classical Indian logic, the

Nyāya, acknowledges three methods of judgement *(pramāṇa)*: the teaching of those who are accepted to be an authority *(āptopadeśa)*, observation *(pratyakṣa)* and inference *(anumāna)*. In another context (*Sūtrasthāna,* XI, 17, 25) a fourth *pramāṇa* is mentioned: the *yukti* which is the rational arrangement leading to a consistent representation of all the facts considered. But this *yukti* does not really constitute a distinct mode of getting information. It is the process that synthesises information.[1] The first method of judgement is defined in the following manner: "*Āptopadeśa* means the word of the authorities. The authorities are those whose knowledge is beyond question, who have an organised and ready memory, and who are observers without joy or sorrow. Their word, owing to their quality, is a proof. By contrast, the word of one who is drunk, insane, stupid, passionate, corrupted or satisfied with himself is not a proof" (*Vimānasthāna,* IV, 4). It is furthermore specified that the teaching of the authorities is the first source of knowledge of the diseases and that observation and inference can only be practised thereafter. Analogy *(upamāna)*, acknowledged as a *pramāṇa* by *Nyāya* and other Indian philosophical schools, is rejected by āyurvedic medicine which knows its deceptive nature in clinical practice. It has nevertheless been made use of by the medical authors but only to facilitate the comprehension of their expositions and not as a method of proof by itself. Another part of the text (*Vimānasthāna,* VIII) gives a series of definitions of terms of logic and reviews the different procedures of discussion designed to make the physicians win in public debates. This importance given to the teaching of logic in medical education testifies to the concern for reasoning processes of the medical circles of ancient India.

There has been much discussion also concerning the relationship between Āyurveda and the philosophical system of *Vaiśeṣika*, notably as regards the medical ideas relating to time. The *Vaiśeṣika* has as its object the study of the special characteristics of things, their *viśeṣa*. The *Vaiśeṣikasūtra*, which constitutes the reference text of this school, dates from the early centuries of the Christian era, but its contents seem to show older interpolations. Time appears therein as one of the nine elementary constituents of Nature and is considered a non-material and eternal substance in contrast to substances that are material and non-eternal which are earth, water, fire and air. It is the cause of the production, preservation and disappearance of all things. This conception is attested in medical literature. We read for example in the corpus of Hārīta:

"Time *(kāla)* incites *(kalayate)* the people, time incites the world... that is why it is called *Kāla*... Time is indeed a blessed god, it is manifestly the supreme Lord. Time is the author of creation, preservation and destruction, and is always the same. By time everything is arranged. That is why it is called *Kāla*... Time emits the elements, time destroys the creatures, time sleeps, is awakened. Yes, time is unsurpassable. In time, the gods perish and in time the Asuras and the Serpent-demons, the kings and all the living beings, in time everything perishes..." (*Hārītasaṃhitā,* I, IV, 9-17).

In this passage, *Kāla* is the supreme divinity described in the *Atharvaveda* and of which one finds a more popular conception in the *Mahābhārata*. The importance given to time figures in the very name of this medical system: Āyurveda. It is the science *(veda)* of the *Āyus*, the "vital time", the "duration of life", a term which one encounters already in the *Veda*s to denote time (cf. for example *Ṛgveda*, X, 17, 4). In āyurvedic medicine, time is also one of the major factors which one must take into account in determining the causes of the disease and in therapy. Indeed, the medical texts abound in dietary and behavioural prescriptions "appropriate to the time" *(kālasātmya)*. In these texts, the term *kāla* denotes both the time "which flows perpetually" *(nityaga)* and the time as a "phase" *(avasthika)* (cf. the definition of the *Carakasaṃhitā, Vimānasthāna*, I, 21). The time "which flows perpetually" is, as the texts tell us, the cycle of the seasons *(saṃvatsara)*. This time is also called *pariṇāma*, "change" (*Carakasaṃhitā*, ibid. VIII, 76). It is an objective time characterised by the succession of the days and the nights and the return of the seasons. The time as a "phase" is related to disease. It is the phases that the patient goes through, or in other words the different "stages of the disease". Here it is a subjective time as perceived by the patient and on which the physician is capable of acting by prescribing a treatment and a diet which are both appropriate to the season and to the state of development of the disease, in order to restore the balance between the patient and his environment. This conception of time is at the root of a certain number of notions which, in Āyurveda, are related to biological rhythms. These notions appear notably in the āyurvedic principles of general and sexual hygiene, dietetics and behaviour. Indeed, Āyurveda has endeavoured to define rules of living and prescribe treatments in harmony with the different rhythms which govern man during his life.

The practical experience of Āyurveda in this area is not at all negligible and deserves to be studied thoroughly in the light of current data on chronobiology.

II. Knowledge of Anatomy

The anatomical nomenclature of Āyurveda is rich, but the notions covered by them are fairly rudimentary, especially as regards visceral anatomy. However, the value of opening corpses was known and the *Suśrutasaṃhitā* (*Śārīrasthāna*, V, 49-56) even describes a procedure of dissection closely resembling a procedure called *hydrotomie* suggested by Lacauchie[2] in the nineteenth century. The Indian procedure consists in letting the corpse decompose in running water for several days, before detaching the different parts by means of a bamboo brush. But, in the absence of sufficient means to prevent putrefaction, such a method could not give satisfactory results. And as the conceptions of the brahmanical moral code were opposed to true methodical dissections of well-preserved corpses, anatomical knowledge remained scanty. Hence, errors and lacunas are numerous in the lists of organs furnished by the ancient medical texts.

Osteology is fairly important in Indian anatomy,[3] but it holds out little interest as regards the constitution of the medical doctrines. The human body is divided into six parts, the two arms, the two legs, the head and the neck, the trunk, between which are distributed the different bones. The *Carakasaṃhitā* lists no less than 360, including the teeth and the nails, but their description and their distribution do not always correspond to anatomical reality. In fact, the number 360 had been fixed from the time of the vedic texts to establish a relationship between the number of bones and that of the days of the year, which was earlier considered as constituted by three hundred and sixty days.

Furthermore, it appears that the muscles were seen as just masses of flesh maintained in place and attached to the skeleton by several hundreds of ligaments ensuring the cohesion of the whole. The *Suśrutasaṃhitā* evaluates their number as 500 and indicates their distribution as well, but this is somewhat fanciful.

The hollow organs or "receptacles" were better known. The stomach is called the "receptacle of the uncooked" while the intestines are the "receptacle of the cooked". The gall bladder is the "receptacle of the bile", while the bladder is of the urine and the uterus of the embryo. Curiously, in the ancient period, each lung seems to have been considered as a different organ, for the *Suśrutasaṃhitā* names the right lung *kloman* and the left *pupphusa*. But the *Carakasaṃhitā* uses only the first term. The heart is described as having the form of an inverted lotus bud. This comparison appears certainly to be based on anatomical observation, for the heart does indeed seem to be suspended from the arch of the aorta, somewhat like a flower bud at the end of a curved stalk. Among these organs, the best described are those on which surgical operations were performed: the rectum, the uterus and the bladder.

Among a great many anatomical formations identified by Āyurveda, the organic vessels deserve special mention. The medical texts know three kinds: the *dhamanī*, the *śirā* and the *srotas*. *Dhamanī* and *śirā* (under the form *hirā*) are already found in a spell from the *Atharvaveda* against hemorrhages, with the precise sense of "blood vessel". The major *dhamanī* are 24 in number which are ramified into several branches:

"Those who go upwards maintain the organism by transporting particular things: sound, contact, taste, odour, inspiration, exhalation, yawning, hunger, laughter, speech, crying, etc. They reach the heart and are trebled, they are (then) thirty. Among them, ten transport, two by two, wind, bile, phlegm, blood and organic juice. By eight, sounds, forms, tastes and odours are grasped. By two, we speak, by two we shout, by two we sleep, by two we wake up. And two carry tears, two which are located in the breasts carry the milk of women..." (*Suśrutasaṃhitā, Śārīrasthāna*, IX, 3-4).

The *śirā* are more numerous and finer than the *dhamanī* and usually only fluids which have little density circulate in them. There are stated to be 700 of them, distributed into four groups of 175, according to the nature of the substances which circulate in them – organic breaths, phlegm, bile or blood. Various colours are attributed to them according to their contents. As regards *srotas*, 22 in number, they denote the vessels opening on the outside like the nostrils, the oesophagus or the windpipe.

The Indian surgeon had above all to know the "vulnerable regions" (*marman*), injury to which is either fatal, or particularly serious. The notion of *marman* goes back to a vedic conception. The word is derived from the root *MṚ*, which means "to die", and denotes above all a lethal point. The classical treatises, which carefully catalogue these bodily zones, describe them as seats of vital energy. They list 107 of them divided into five categories according to their location (flesh, vessels, ligaments, bones, joints) and into five categories, according to the seriousness of the harm resulting from injuries to them. The details given by the texts enable us to locate them fairly easily. They are anatomical reference points corresponding most often to big vessel-nerve bundles, tendons or important nerve ganglia, injuries to which are serious because of hemorrhage, paralysis or disabilities that they cause. Subsequently, these notions were developed in the "therapeutics of the vital zones" *(marmacikitsā)* which constitutes a speciality of Siddha medicine.

III. Representations of the Vital Functions

In the āyurvedic system, the totality of the transformations undergone by the seven organic substances (*dhātu*) is governed by the combined play and balance of wind, fire and water, present and active in the body in the form of three other elements. Indeed, wind, the essential motive force of the Universe, is also that of the body in which it is represented by the ßvital breathû or *prāṇa*, which also plays a very important role in the conception and practices of yoga. "Fire" is represented by a principle which collects in the form of "bile" or *pitta*. As regards water, it is found in the form of *kapha* or *śleṣman*, "phlegm", a substance common to all the bodily serous fluids and secretions. Each of these three principles acts by assuming five secondary forms which correspond to the different vital functions and manifestations. Their action works towards a complex and autonomous process of balancing which maintains the organism (by the constant renewal of its constituents) and in good health. These Indian ideas are very close to the notion of homeostasis, already anticipated by Claude Bernard during the last century and which Walter Cannon (1871-1945) described as the totality of organic processes which act to maintain the stationary state of the organism, in its morphology and in its internal conditions, despite external disturbances.

The organic wind is subdivided into a "frontal breath" (the actual *prāṇa*) which is responsible for respiration and swallowing, and which sustains the body; an "upward breath" (*udāna*), which produces speech; a "concentrated breath" (*samāna*), present in the stomach and the intestines, which stirs up the bodily fire ensuring digestion and assimilation of foods; a "diffused breath" (*vyāna*) which ensures the circulation of the fluids and the movements of the members; lastly a "downward breath" (*apāna*) which expels the excrements (*Suśrutasaṃhitā*, Nidānasthāna, I, 4-12).

The fiery principle is represented by the "cooking fire" *(pācaka-agni)* which consumes foods and maintains the body warm, the "colouring fire" *(rañjaka-agni)* which reddens the *rasa* to transform it into blood, the "accomplishing fire" *(sādhaka-agni)* which awakens the desires in the heart, the "seer" *(ālocaka)* which ensures vision, and the "illuminating fire" *(bhrājaka-agni)* which confers to the complexion its radiance (*Suśrutasaṃhitā*, Sūtrasthāna, XXI, 7-13).

The *śleṣman* is located first and foremost in the stomach which serves as a centre for its functions. In the chest, it serves as an element of cohesion and sustains the heart. On the tongue and in the throat, it enables one to perceive the tastes. In the head, it facilitates the sensory faculties. Lastly the *śleṣman* that is found in the joints ensures their perfect articulation (*Suśrutasaṃhitā*, Sūtrasthāna, XV, 5; XXI, 15).

These few examples show how inadequate the usual translations of *pitta* and *śleṣman* into "bile" and "phlegm" are. We have retained them for want of a better translation, but it must never be forgotten that *pitta* and *śleṣman* denote altogether different things from bile and phlegm as they are commonly understood.

Of these three principles, it is the organic wind, under its different forms, which is considered as the most important vital element. According to the *Carakasaṃhitā* (Sūtrasthāna,XII, 8), "it is the promoter of movements of all kinds. It restrains and guides the mind. It activates all the faculties, and helps in the enjoyment of their objects, distributes all the elements *(dhātu)* of the organism, gives consistency to the body, promotes speech. It is the substance of contact *(sparśa)* and of sound *(śabda)*, the basis of hearing *(śrotra)* and of touch *(sparśana)*, the source of joy and liveliness, the kindler of fire... ". It therefore ensures by its action the ingestion, digestion and assimilation of food, the differentiation of the organic substances and their distribution, as well as the internal circulation of the fluids, respiration and general motivity, covering in this way a number of aspects of functioning attributed to the central, peripheral and autonomous nervous systems.

In such a system, digestion compared to cooking of the foods by the *pācaka* fire, stirred up by the *samāna* breath. The chyle *(rasa)* which results from this cooking constitutes the essential substance of the organism, from which all the other substances are developed in the course of successive transformations. The waste (*mala*) which results from the transformation of the foods constitutes the faeces and the urine. Those which result from the differentiation of the *dhātus* form the "phlegm" and the "bile" (respectively considered as by-products of the *rasa* and the blood) as well as the earwax, the nasal mucus, the sweat, the hair, the nails, etc. (*Carakasaṃhitā,* Cikitsāsthāna, XV, 18-19).

The seven *dhātu*s contain a liquid principle which makes them alive and which is named *ojas*, that is to say "strength". It is located in the heart, and the breaths which are supported by it distribute it into the whole of the body through certain vessels. According to Caraka the *ojas* is produced by the semen, but Suśruta indicates that all the *dhātu*s contribute to its formation. "By the strength which is in it, the flesh is firm and developed, there is ease in all the movements, clarity of voice and of complexion, the external and internal organs fulfill their own functions" (*Suśrutasaṃhitā*, Sūtrasthāna, XV, 24).

Āyurveda considers the heart as a very important organ, both the seat of awareness and the principal receptacle of *rasa*, blood and *ojas*. It is also the heart which is responsible for the distribution of these three fluids in the entire body, by means of numerous organic ducts which end there. But its true function was not known to the ancient texts.

The data concerning respiratory physiology are very rudimentary. Respiration is one of the functions of the *prāṇa* which is thought to take the inspired air up to the heart after passing through the windpipe. Śārṅgadhara, in the thirteenth or fourteenth century, describes the heart as the principal seat of "air". He however indicates that the *udāna* breath is found in the lungs. He tells us also that after having passed through the inside of the heart, the *prāṇa* breath goes out to gorge itself with the nectar of air and enters afresh into the body to nourish it and to maintain the digestive fire. The presence of water vapour in the expired air did not go unnoticed. It is no doubt why Caraka observes that the lung (*kloman*) is the root of the canals which conduct the water. Unfortunately this observation remained insufficiently developed and the physicians contented themselves with inaccurate and arbitrary conjectures on the role of the major organs.

IV. Psychological Conceptions

Psychological conceptions play a fundamental role in the teachings of Āyurveda. The connection between the body and the mind is asserted in the most direct manner by the Sanskrit medical texts: "The body is governed by the psyche and the psyche by the body" (*Carakasaṃhitā*, Śārīrasthāna, IV, 36).

This importance given to the body–mind unity appears in the very definition of life according to Āyurveda. Indeed, in this system, life is seen at once as a "psychological continuum" (*cetanānuvṛtti*), a "support" (*dhāri*) of the body, a "vital phenomenon (*jīvita*), a "permanent process" (*nityaga*) and a factor of "continuity" (*anubandha*), throughout the successive lives of the psychic being (*Carakasaṃhitā*, Sūtrasthāna, I, 42), death being just the loss of the "gross body" (*sthūlaśarīra*) whose constituents are perishable.

It is interesting to note that, according to Āyurveda, the psyche represents the contribution of the previous existences of the incorporated soul. This is entirely in conformity with the Indian theory of *karman*. The word *karman*, derived from the root *KṚ*, "to do", means "deed", "action", but denotes also the results of the good and bad actions in the form of merit or demerit, the inexorable consequence of acts accomplished in previous lives. A whole theory has been developed around *karman* which has become a central dogma of Hinduism, Buddhism and Jainism, among others. By affecting the *sūkṣmaśarīra* or "subtle body", or in other words the psychic individual, the Self (*ātman*), the permanent and unconscious substratum of the human being (*sattva*), *karman* obliges him indefinitely to undergo a new birth in a human or other form, determined by the quality of his past acts.

According to the learned conception of *karman*, the acts, as well as the thoughts and the desires accumulated in the course of each existence, leave traces in the psyche which are called "*vāsanā*" (literally "perfume" to denote their subtle nature) and which, organised into subconscious clusters, the *saṃskāra* (which may be superficially compared with the "complexes" of the psychology of the subconscious), determine the innate tendencies of each individual.

The sensory functions (*indriya*) are put in relation with the five major elements. Vision proceeds from fire, hearing from space, smell from earth, taste from water and touch from air. The centralisation and coordination of sensory data, carried by the "wind", the "bile" and the "phlegm", as well as the development of ideas take place in the *manas* (from *MAN*, "to think") which the texts describe as the central psychic organ.

The vessels described as white in colour probably denote the nerves. The inclusion of the nervous system in the vascular system is explained perhaps by the fact that the authors of the classical treatises considered the heart to be the seat of consciousness. It must nevertheless be noted that another author, Bhela, places the *manas* in the head. He however distinguishes it from the organ of awareness, or *citta*, which he locates in the heart, according to the usual theory of medical works.

The observation of the relationship between the body and the mind has led the Indian physicians to notions of personal temperament and physiognomy. āyurvedic biotypology is based on two criteria, one constitutive, the other psychological. The first typology describes three kinds of temperaments based on the predominance of one of the three vital principles: the "windy, the "bilious", the "phlegmatic". The second typological system of Āyurveda categorises the individuals according to the properties (*guṇa*) of the mind. The ideal standard of behaviour is that which corresponds to a predominance of *sattva*, "purity", according to the *Sāṃkhya* philosophy.

But it is above all in yoga circles that the most interest was shown for the psyche. This Indian discipline of control over the body and the mind comprises several stages whose final goal is the liberation from the cycle of births, the *saṃsāra*. To obtain this result, the practitioner must endeavour to reach a special state of awareness, a "fourth" (*turīya*) state, which transcends the three conditions of wakefulness, dream, and profound sleep. This state is necessary, according to yoga, for the final good frame of mind of the transmigrating human being to accede to deliverance (*mokṣa*).

V. Diseases and Pathology

According to Āyurveda, diseases (*roga*, *vyādhi*) are of two kinds, exogenous and endogenous. The former are due to accidental causes (blows, injuries, bites, falls, burns, etc.). All the others result from an "imbalance of the *dhātu*s" (*dhātuvaiṣamya*), or in other words disturbances in the normal balance of the elements which constitute the substance of the body and which animate it. "Wind, bile and phlegm, in the normal state, enable a man to have a long life, with his faculties intact, endowed with vigour, good appearance, and health... But, if they become abnormal, they lead him to great adversity..." (*Carakasaṃhitā*, Sūtrasthāna, XII, 14). That is why this triad of vital elements has been given the name of *tridoṣa*, the "three disorders".

The conditions of perturbation of their functions are complex in most cases. The alteration of just one of these elements or just one of its secondary forms can unleash a disease by virtue of the disturbances resulting in the functioning of the others. Often two among them or even all three of them are simultaneously involved, in varying degrees, in the production of different ailments. Hence there is a very large number of pathogenic combinations. The *Carakasaṃhitā* distinguishes 62 types, according to the number, nature and the degree of excitation of the perturbed elements, and follows it up by a list of clinical symptoms which enable one to recognise in a patient the type of pathogenic combination responsible for the disease. For example, the excitation of the *samāna* breath produces illnesses such as various kinds of tumours, diarrhoea, dysuria and constipation. But when the *samāna* is combined with bile, there is sweating, inflammation and fainting fits.

The perturbations of "wind", "bile" and "phlegm" can in their turn affect the other *dhātu*s, the joints or the vascular system. The elements, the tissues and the organs interact, and imbalance of the ones lead to imbalance of the others. It is thus that the blood, a vital fluid in its normal state, can become the seat or source of various illnesses, consequent upon an imbalance which affects it directly or through the agency of the *doṣa*s.[4] For example, the excited "wind" which has reached the blood can provoke ulcers, "that which resides in the flesh, painful protuberances and, similarly, that which resides in the fat, indolent non-ulcerous protuberances. That which has arrived in the vessels can produce shooting pain, contraction and fullness of the vessels" (*Suśrutasaṃhitā*, Nidānasthāna, I, 25-76). When it reaches the sinews (*snāyu*), it results in paralysis or convulsions. Reaching the joints, it makes them painful and swollen. It is also responsible for the cracking of the bones. "Contaminated" blood can block the path of "wind" which, becoming excited by this blockage, can inordinately disturb the blood. One then speaks of "wind–blood". The heating up of the blood following excitation of "bile" gives rise to the clinical hemorrhagical forms called *raktapitta*, "blood-bile". Under this name are covered all the illnesses which result in a loss of blood or of "blood with bile" through the openings of the body: haematemesis, haemoptysis, melaena, nosebleeds, etc. The combined action of "wind" and "bile" on the blood provokes inflammation of the feet. The simultaneous disturbance in "wind" and "phlegm" causes people to be inactive, dumb or to stammer. Finally some serious forms of diseases are attributed to the combination of the three *doṣa*s.

Some parallels have often been drawn between these ideas and some of the data from Greek medicine. The text *Airs* of the Hippocratic Collection describes notably a pathology by the association of the blood and the "wind", which does bring to mind the theory of the *Suśrutasaṃhitā* relating to the pathogenic role of "wind–blood". Furthermore, there exists a remarkable analogy between the doctrine of the *tridoṣa* and a theory described by Plato at the end of his *Timaeus*. Even though the priority of the Greek texts cannot be disputed, the hypothesis of a Greek influence on the formation of Āyurveda cannot be accepted for explaining these concordances, for the āyurvedic conceptions go back by their origins to an epoch that is much earlier than that of the formation of the Greek medical schools. On the other hand, the communication of the Indian ideas to certain Greek medical circles is attested by the mention of āyurvedic drugs under their Indian names in Greek texts.

The perturbations in the functions of "wind", "bile" and "phlegm" are themselves related to multiple causes called *nidāna* which are looked for mainly in the behaviour of the patient, his food, having regard to the external circumstances, climatic or fortuitous. Thus, "among the people with delicate health, among those who eat and behave improperly, consequent on excessive fatigue due to women, wines and exercises, consequent on affliction, consequent on deviation from the diet of the season and the unbridled use of fatty substances, etc. wind–blood is excited in the continent man as well as in the corpulent man" (*Suśrutasaṃhitā*, Nidānasthāna, I, 39-40). The normal activity of "wind" is modified notably by excess exercise, prolonged wakefulness, long horse rides, walking, a diet rich in spicy, hot, sour or caustic foods, or by cloudy or rainy weather. Fear, anger, fatty foods, fermented drinks and heat perturb the "bile". Finally, lack of exercise, laziness, immoderate use of certain cereals, meals at close intervals and wintry weather harm the proper functioning of the "phlegm".

Dietary deviations are often criticised. The *Carakasaṃhitā* teaches that he who stuffs himself with oily, sweet, heavy, and fatty foods, with cereals, wine, flesh of the animals of the marshes or aquatic animals, milk and its derivatives, sugar, and flour-based preparations, and who at the same time abstains from physical exercise... will suffer illnesses provoked by satiety. Among these illnesses, Āyurveda categorises urinary affections, urticaria, pruritis, fever, leprosy, stomach troubles, dysuria, anorexia, fatigue, impotence, obesity, feelings of heaviness in the body, obstructions in the organs and the channels of the senses. Some of these illnesses: fever, anorexia, dysuria can also be caused by undernourishment which is capable of provoking cough, *costal* pains, constipation, and in some cases insanity and delirium.

The section of the *Carakasaṃhitā* devoted to etiology treats successively the "occasions of production" (*nidāna*) of fevers (*jvara*), hemorrhagic maladies (*raktapitta*), internal tumours (*gulma*), urinary alterations (*prameha*), dermatoses (*kuṣṭha*), consumptive maladies (*śoṣa*), mental illnesses (*unmāda*) and epilepsy (*apasmāra*). The corresponding section of

Suśrutasaṃhitā is more important. It contains 16 chapters which treat most of the same affections and tackles in addition the etiology of a certain number of localised illnesses such as hemorrhoids, anal fistulas, erysipelas, swellings (hernias, hydroceles...), as well as affections of the mouth. Suśruta does not confine himself to a simple exposition of the causes of the illnesses; he also gives, or repeats, in these chapters, the physiological theories which are at the root of the pathogenic hypotheses of Āyurveda.

The etiology of mental illness described under the name *unmāda* (insanity) also assigns a role to two other specific dosas of the psyche: *rajas* and *tamas*. They are two of the three components of the *prakṛti* according to *Sāṃkhya* philosophy. *Rajas*, which represents activity, is at the root of desires and passions. When it dominates the character of an individual, he is full of himself, loquacious, angry, and seeks competition. *Tamas* connotes ignorance and lethargy. A subject who has predominant "tamasic" tendencies is fearful and sad. Confusion prevails in his mind. The accentuation of these tendencies can become pathological. Such pathogenic theories exclude hypotheses of a demoniacal agency in the production of illnesses. All the same the belief in demons was too prevalent not to be introduced into scholarly medicine and it accepted, in certain cases of "possession", the action of supernatural beings as the cause of profound changes in the personality of the patient who adopts the type of behaviour attributed to one or other of these beings. But, according to Āyurveda, these entities do not act directly, they only complicate the natural morbid states corresponding, according to the psychiatrists who have studied them, to hysterical manifestations or psychotic dissociations.[5]

Nosology is highly developed. It categorises the diseases sometimes according to their supposed origin, sometimes according to the nature of their symptoms. The *Suśrutasaṃhitā* (Sūtrasthāna, XXIV, 4-11), for example, distinguishes three major categories of diseases subdivided into several classes: those which have their origin in the body, those due to external causes and those due to providential causes. The first category comprises hereditary and congenital diseases or those which were supposed to be such, as well as diseases produced by the *doṣa*s. Among the hereditary diseases Suśruta categorises leprosy and hemorrhoids. They can be inherited either from the father or from the mother. Among the congenital diseases figure blindness, deafness and the monstrosities attributed either to a disturbance of the *rasa*, or to "an unsatisfied desire or a fault of the pregnant woman". Those produced by the *doṣa*s may be physical or mental. The second category is reserved to the exogenous diseases. They are essentially traumas: injuries caused by weapons, bites of wild animals, insect bites, etc. Lastly, in the last category are grouped the diseases attributed to the change of seasons, maladies of supernatural origin, and those which result from a natural process like old age.

We also find them divided in another way, according to whether they affect the chyle, the blood, the flesh, the fat, the bones, the marrow or the semen. Among the diseases of the chyle are grouped indigestion, jaundice, cachexia and the falling out of hair. The diseases of the blood cover notably erysipelas, abscesses, tumours and hemorrhoids. Diseases of the skin, the head, the mouth, the eyes, etc. are also distinguished. Fevers, which form a group of diseases characterised by the common symptom of hyperthermia, are differentiated according to the action ascribed to the three *doṣa*s and to their combinations in the secondary symptoms which accompany them. The later texts, notably those of Vāgbhaṭa, Mādhava and Cakrapāṇidatta, give us also very elaborate classifications of the diseases, which generally agree in their broad features with that of Suśruta, differing from it only on points of detail. The affections which are categorised under the item *unmāda* are variably classified depending on the authors. As many as 28 varieties are enumerated which correspond broadly to the manic-depressive and schizophrenic psychoses.

In Siddha medicine, the interpretation of the pathological phenomena is founded in part on a system of representation of anatomy and physiology which is not that of classical Āyurveda, but which is found in haṭhayoga and in tantrism. This system, which has also influenced Tibetan medicine, gives major importance to a certain number of "centres" situated in specific regions of the body. These centres, called *cakra* (circles) or *padma* (lotus), the *muṭiccu* or "nodes" of the Tamil texts, are considered as the principal crossroads of the organic breaths. Some coincide moreover with organs which are, according to classical Āyurveda, the seats of vital energy. Hence the correspondences between the different organic functions and the elements of Nature (*prakṛti*), earth, water, fire, air and space. The most important *cakra*s are six in number:

i. The *mūlādhāra* or "support of the base" is located in the recto-genital region. It is connected to the *apāna* breath, smell and locomotion.
ii. The *svādhiṣṭhāna* or "seat of the Self", situated a little above the preceding *cakra*, is connected to taste and to prehension.
iii. The *maṇipūra* or "citadel of the jewel", located in the region of the navel, governs the *samāna* breath and vision.
iv. The *anāhata*, literally the "unbeaten" (so named by allusion to the sound produced by the heart), situated in the region of the heart, is associated with *prāṇa* breath and to touch.
v. The *viśuddha*, the "purified", is located at the throat. It is associated with *udāna* breath, hearing and the mouth.
vi. The *ājñā-cakra* or "centre of command", placed in the head, at the level of the point between the eyebrows, is the seat of mental faculties where the messages of the senses are received and from where the orders to the motor organs are transmitted, hence its name.

Several authors, Indian and Western, have endeavoured to discover the anatomical substratum of these centres, identifying them at times with the sympathetic plexuses. Others think that the identification of the *cakras* with bodily organs is not well-founded. The basis of the descriptions of the *cakras* given in the texts would only be the internal vision of the yogis. It could not also be otherwise since, in addition, the structures in question are not at all anatomical but are situated in the 'subtle body', the *sūkṣmaśarīra*, the permanent foundation of the mental aspect of the person.

All the *cakras* are connected to each other by a system of channels or *nāḍī* which are the paths taken by the breaths circulating in the body. There are supposed to be thousands of them but the majority of the texts generally enumerate only about ten, with their own variants depending on the lists. From among these ten, there are three whose knowledge is essential for the adepts of yoga: *iḍā*, *piṅgalā* and *suṣumnā*. Finally, of these three, *suṣumnā* is the principal one, and all the others are subordinate to it.

The *suṣumnā* is an axial *nāḍī* which rises from the base of the spinal column to the top of the skull. *Iḍā* and *piṅgalā* are lateral vessels which start at the base of the trunk and interwine around the *suṣumnā*, like the serpents round the staff of Caduceus, to reach respectively the left and right nostrils.

In such a system, disease is described as the consequence of an improper circulation of *prāṇa* through the *nāḍīs* saturated with impurities. It is the case, indeed, that the blocking or stagnation of the vital breath in a *nāḍī* produces an imbalance which in turn affects the *dhātus* and causes different ailments according to a process from then on identical with those supposed by the pathogenic theories of Āyurveda. Hence the importance accorded to the yogic techniques of "breath control", "*prāṇāyāma*", both as a preventive method as well as a therapeutic method.

VI. Diagnosis and Prognosis

To identify an ailment, to know its stage of development as well as the part which should be ascribed to each *doṣa* in its production, the āyurvedic practitioner must undertake a minute examination not only of the body of the patient but also of his mental state. The methods of examination must bring into play all the doctor's senses. He must inspect the appearance of the skin, the tongue, the excrement and the shape and the size of the wounds or swellings. He must listen to the sound of the respiration, the *borborygmi* (intestinal rumblings), the cracking of the joints, and pay attention to possible alterations of the voice of the patient. He must also palpate him to evaluate his temperature and the state of his skin. He must also smell the odours emanating from the patient, from his wounds or from his secretions.

The practice of the examination of the pulse, common today in āyurvedic medicine, does not seem to have appeared before the eighth century. The idea of examining the pulse might have been borrowed from China, but the technique attested in India is different and what one expects to learn out of this examination is not what the Chinese physicians look for. Indeed, by taking the pulse the Indian physician claims to recognise the disturbances in the equilibrium of the three vital principles, "wind", "bile" and "phlegm" and in this way he diagnoses all the ailments. The interpretation of the various pulses is connected therefore to the āyurvedic theory of the *tridoṣa*.

The palpation is done by bringing the tips of the index finger, the middle finger and the ring finger close to each other and applying them on the radial artery of the right wrist for men, and the left wrist for women. The texts distinguish several types of pulse according to the amplitude of the pulsation (strong, weak or very weak pulse), the frequency (regular, rapid or slow pulse) and the temperature (hot or cold pulse), whose variations are presumed to reflect the activities of the three *doṣa*s. A pulse which resembles that of a leech or of a snake is considered as indicating excessive activity of "wind". The excitation of "bile" is reflected by beats which recall the jump of a frog or the flight of the crow. The pulse corresponding to an excitation of the "phlegm" is compared to a turtledove. An intermittent pulse signifies a morbid state related to the action of two *doṣa*s. The terminologies of Wang shu-he and Galen are sometimes of the same kind. The Chinese texts mention for example a "frog's leap" pulse. Galen, for his part, speaks of the leap of a goat or of the tail of a mouse. But we must expect to find such analogies in the works that treat pulse.[6] They do not necessarily prove a borrowing from Chinese or from Galenic medicine.

The various examinations are complemented by questioning the patient and his family circle. The purpose of this questioning is not only for the physician to gain information about the circumstances in which the first symptoms appeared and the development of the ailment, but also about the personality of the patient, his activities, his food and his appetite, having regard to the season, the climate and, of course, the psychological context in which the sickness began. The *Carakasaṃhitā* indicates that the patient should also be questioned about his dreams.

All this information enables the physician to determine, in the light of his experience, what elements of the vital functioning accepted by theory are involved. For example, loss of appetite, indigestion, nausea, anemia and a burning sensation are supposed to be the result of a decrease in the activity of the "wind". Dizziness accompanied by pain, cramps and shivering is attributed to a slowing down of the functions of the "phlegm" and to an excess of activity of the "wind" and the "bile". There are long lists of symptoms drawn up in this manner in the Sanskrit medical texts which enable the physician to go back by inference to the root of the ailment. Once the ailment is identified and its causes recognised, it remains for the practitioner to establish a prognosis and to decide on the course of action to put the functions back in order.

In ancient times, the establishment of the prognosis concerning the curability or the incurability of a disease depended more often on divining art than on medical science. Thus, one claimed to foretell the outcome of a disease according to the language, the clothes and the attitude of the messenger who came to fetch the doctor, or else according to the direction of the wind blowing at his arrival, or else according to the dreams of the patient. The anomalies that may be noticed in the sensations of the patient were generally regarded as bad signs (*ariṣṭa*). Other fatal indications could be drawn from the change in his complexion. It is also said that the diseases which affect a Brahmin versed in the Veda, or a king, or a woman, or a child, or an old man, or a timid person, or the servant of a king, or a deceitful man, or a man who hides his disease, or a man who has no control over his senses, or a man in extreme poverty or a man who has no one to care for him, can develop into an incurable form (*Suśrutasaṃhitā*, Sūtrasthāna, X, 7).

But even in the use of physiognomy or the interpretation of dreams the scientific spirit of Āyurveda asserts its rights. The *Carakasaṃhitā* gives for example the following explanation concerning the prognostic value of dreams announcing death: they are hallucinations provoked by the *doṣa*s which affect the channels which are vectors of the sensory impressions to the mind. These dreams are therefore to be interpreted as serious signs, because they are themselves produced by serious disorders.

NOTES

1. Concerning this notion of *yukti*, see P. S. Filliozat, Yukti, le quatriẸme pramāṇa des médecins (*Carakasaṃhitā*, Sūtrasthāna, XI, 25), *Journal of the European Ayurvedic Society*, I, 1990, pp.33-46.

2. Traité d'Hydrotomie ou Injections d'eau Continue dans les Recherches Anatomiques by A.E. Lacauchie, P. BailliẸre (1853).

3. See the work of A.F.R. Hoernle, *Studies in the Medicine of Ancient India*, Part I, Osteology or the bones of the human body, Oxford, Clarendon Press, 1907 (reprint, New York, AMS Press, 1978).

4. See G. Mazars, Le sang et les plantes du sang dans la médecine âyurvédique, *Savoirs, matériaux pour une anthropologie des savoirs, no. 1: Les plantes, le sang*, 1988, pp. 149-157.

5. H. Stork, Principes de base des traitements psychiatriques dans l'âyurveda, *Scientia Orientalis*, 16, 1979, p. 25.

6. Cf. M.D. Grmek, Les reflets de la sphygnologie chinoise dans la médecine occidentale, *La biologie médicale*, numéro hors série, février 1962, pp. XLVIII-L.

CHAPTER 3

PREVENTIVE MEDICINE

Of all the ancient medicines, it is probably āyurvedic medicine which, from its origins, has accorded the greatest importance to hygiene, to diet, to physical exercises and to massage, both as means of prevention and as curative methods. The rules of hygiene and of diet were already extremely numerous and elaborate in the treatises of Caraka and Suśruta who devote several chapters to them. These rules take into account not only the climate, the season and the circumstances, but also the temperament of each individual.

I. Hygiene and Life Style

One of the most elementary requirements was that of bathing. According to the *Suśrutasaṃhitā*, the bath removes somnolence, heating up and fatigue; it fights thirst, itching and sweating; it is depurative, purifies the sense organs, clarifies the blood and stimulates the digestive fire. It must not be too cold in winter, or too hot in summer, and must not be taken immediately after a meal. It is inadvisable to bathe in case of fever, diarrhoea, headaches, indigestion or sickness due to a disturbance of the "wind".

Great importance is also attached to oral hygiene which comprises cleaning the teeth, scraping the tongue and rinsing the mouth. The teeth are cleaned using a short stick from one of the following plant species: *Pongamia pinnata* Pier., *Nerium indicum* Mill., *Calotropis gigantea* (L.) R. Br., *Aganosma dichotoma* (Roth) K. Schum. or *Terminalia tomentosa* W. & A., one of whose extremities is crushed to expose its fibres. For the tongue a curved metallic scraper is used.

Several old texts recommended chewing regularly a certain number of aromatic substances, such as nutmeg (*Myristica fragrans* Houtt.), arecanut (fruit of the *Areca Catechu* L.), cubeb (*Piper cubeba* L.), clove (*Eugenia caryophyllata,* Thunb.) or betel leaf (*Piper betle* L.), at the beginning of the day and at the end of meals, to perfume the breath or because of their stimulating or digestive properties. Betel, which is so widely chewed in India, is generally made up of pieces of arecanut, a fresh betel leaf and a certain quantity of quicklime. It is the combination of these three components that confers to the betel its particularly pleasant taste. Sometimes catechu and camphor are added to it. The chewing of betel not only has the effect of perfuming the breath, but also constitutes a very mild stimulant leading to a feeling of wellbeing. The *Hārītasaṃhitā* says that it is "an aphrodisiac, a purifier, makes the voice rich, is good for the throat, is an appetiser and a cough mixture".

The *Carakasaṃhitā* gives also the recipe for nasal drops to be used during the rainy season, in autumn and in summer, to prevent a certain number of ailments: stiff neck, headaches, rhinitis. Finally, there was use of collyriums, perfumes and cosmetic products of all kinds.

Prescriptions concerning general and sexual hygiene are also given by the texts of sexology which India has elevated to the rank of a true science. The oldest text which has come down to us, and the most important, is the *Kāmasūtra* or "Aphorisms on pleasure" of Vātsyāyana, which may go back to the fourth or the fifth century. The author describes in it the everyday grooming of the man of fashion. The last section of the treatise proposes aesthetic and medical formulas.

Sanskrit haṭhayoga texts also give an important place to body hygiene. Side by side with general hygiene, haṭhayoga prescribes special purification techniques for the body known under the name of *ṣaṭkarman*, literally the "six actions". According to the *Haṭhayogapradīpikā* (II, 21), they are addressed only to those who suffer from an excess of fat or "phlegm":

i. *Dhauti*, internal cleansing, consists in swallowing slowly then regurgitating a long strip of cloth soaked in warm water. This cleansing is supposed to have the effect of curing cough, breathlessness, enlargement of the spleen, leprosy and some twenty-odd ailments caused by an improper functioning of "phlegm".

ii. *Basti*, enema, is carried out by aspirating water through the rectum. This is an operation whose mechanism is disputed: either voluntary control of the smooth muscular fibres or, as seems more in conformity with the classical data, the action of the small intestines and of the muscles of the abdominal wall, acting on the rectum like on a bulb made of rubber.

iii. *Neti* denotes the washing of the nose. It consists in introducing a long thread soaked in oil through a nostril and drawing it out through the mouth. It is supposed to cure all the ailments "which appear in the part of the body situated above the collar bones", in other words all the ocular, oto-rhino-laryngological and odonto-stomatological affections.

iv. *Trāṭaka* is an exercise of ocular concentration which is believed to cure maladies of the eye. It consists of fixing the gaze, without blinking the eyes, on a very small object, like the incandescent tip of an incense stick, until tears start flowing. In reality, the subject suffering from an ocular ailment is not capable of doing this and is taken for someone who has not sufficiently pursued the treatment. By contrast, when the patient is recovering, the exercise can be done in the normal way. Therefore in this specific case a test of recovery is mistakenly believed to be a therapy.[1]

v. *Nauli* is a rolling movement imparted to the stomach by the alternate contraction of the side muscles of the abdomen.

vi. *Kapālabhāti* denotes the action of breathing at a very rapid pace. This ventilation is supposed to dry up all the ailments attributed to "phlegm".

II. Yoga and Remedial Gymnastics

In the chapters relating to prevention, the *Carakasaṃhitā* (Sūtrasthāna, VII, 31-34) emphasizes the benefits of physical exercises (*dehavyāyāma*). It is said there that gymnastics makes the body light, increases its capacity for work, diminishes the *doṣa*s and stimulates the "digestive fire". But it must be practised with moderation. Today, āyurvedic medicine is readily complemented by haṭhayoga exercises and there exist in India a good many hospitals and dispensaries where traditional physicians, physicians trained in modern methods and teachers of yoga cooperate in treating the patients. It is often through the study of haṭhayoga that many Westerners learn of Indian traditional medicine. In fact, there exist close connections between this medicine and the traditions of yoga. Indeed, yoga exercises constitute before all else a totality of techniques that put into practice the physiological and psychological theories developed in āyurvedic circles.

The practice of yoga presupposes a healthy body. Hence it is not a therapy in the proper sense of the term. Nevertheless, various yoga schools have claimed to prevent and even treat diseases by means of the techniques that they have developed. The haṭhayoga manuals that have come down to us indeed lay emphasis on techniques and experiments with a prophylactic or curative aim. The best known among these manuals are the *Haṭhayogapradīpikā*, the *Gherandasaṃhitā* and the *Śivasaṃhitā*, probably written towards the end of the medieval period. It is to be noted that their authors belonged to movements or schools which had connections with circles of alchemists and physicians. Svātmārāma, the redactor of the *Haṭhayogapradīpikā*, describes himself as a disciple of the Siddhas.

Thus, many of the postures and the breathing exercises associated with them were thought to prevent or cure all kinds of diseases. It is said, for example, in the *Haṭhayogapradīpikā* (I, 27), that the posture known as Matsyendra (name of a legendary master) stimulates the "digestive fire" and breaks the circle of diseases. Another posture, that of dorsal extension or *paścimottānāsana,*[2] facilitates the circulation of the "vital breath" at the back of the body and is thought to rekindle the "digestive fire". As another example, we may cite the breathing technique denoted by the name of *śītalī*, "the refresher", which is supposed to combat simultaneously the harmful effects of "bile" (*pitta*), swellings, splenomegaly and fevers. For this one must breathe in, with the mouth open, lips rounded, by sticking out the tongue a little, in such a way that the aspirated air produces a whistle.

This aspect of the practice of haṭhayoga has led several authors to talk of "yogic medicine", of "yoga therapy" or even to describe haṭhayoga as a form of medicine distinct from the other traditional medicines of India. In fact, the Indian beliefs concerning the preventive or curative effects of haṭhayoga are not entirely unfounded. They can be explained, partially at least, by the rather exceptional character of the physiological effects of the haṭhayoga exercises, which scientific investigations of recent decades have enabled us to appreciate. The earliest studies of interest are those of Dr. Thérèse Brosse who, as early as in 1936, was able to establish the physiological effects of some of the practices of haṭhayoga, from simultaneous recordings of pulse, respiration and electrocardiogram done on yogis in India itself.[3] Many other studies have since been made and a certain number of medical applications of yoga have already been studied or suggested by doctors or by physiologists. Unfortunately, there have not yet been truly comprehensive studies by simultaneous investigations of all the elements of each exercise in the same subject. Very often, moreover, the exercises studied are not rigorously identified and described in relation to the classical treatises of haṭhayoga which define them and which specify their modalities and their duration. Finally, these studies are confined to recordings and dosages, and do not take into account the overall psychological dimension of the experiences that are studied.

In any case, yoga does not constitute an independent medical system. The notions of hygiene and dietetics incorporated in the teaching of haṭhayoga are not peculiar to it. They have been mentioned in the oldest Sanskrit medical texts. Similarly, the elementary notions of physiology and pathology to which haṭhayoga texts allude are those of classical Āyurveda.

III. Food and Dietetics

In the *Carakasaṃhitā*, a lot of information concerning food is grouped together in the four chapters which constitute the *Annapānacatuṣka*, the "tetrad concerning food and drinks". In Suśruta's treatise, food is treated in chapters XX and XLV of the first part. We also find interesting indications in other parts of these two treatises, notably in the chapters devoted to life style and therapeutics. Another instructive work, despite its late compilation, is the *Hārītasaṃhitā* whose teachings, especially in the areas of hygiene and dietetics, complement those of the classical tradition represented by the collections of Caraka and Suśruta. According to these authors, the nutritive value of foods depends on their properties (*guṇa*), which are related to the basic elements (earth, water, fire, air and space) which predominate in it. Thus the savour of foods plays a great role in food prescriptions. It is said for example that sweet (*madhura*) foods enrich the blood, the marrow and the sperm. Sour (*amla*) foods stimulate the digestive functions. As regards those which are bitter (*tikta*), they sharpen the appetite, etc. This importance given to food flows from the conceptions of Āyurveda relating to the vital functioning and to its perturbations, conceptions which have facilitated the development of an elaborate dietetics testifying to a great concern for adaptation to the climates and to the populations of India. Practical experience and observations accumulated during the course of the centuries have manifestly played a decisive role in the development of this dietetics, whose rules have been sought to be justified from established doctrines.[4]

The oldest Sanskrit texts lay stress on the importance of a well-balanced diet, both from the quantitative and the qualitative points of view. According to the *Carakasaṃhitā*, the quantity of food depends on the capacity of digestion (*agnibala*, literally "strength of the fire"), so much so that even foods considered as very easy to digest must not be consumed in excessive quantities. It is also said that even a starving individual should be careful not to consume too much food, precisely because, in his case, the "digestive fire" is weakened.

The medical texts systematically enumerate all varieties of edible products indicating their different properties, according to the temperament, behaviour and state of health of each individual, having regard also to the season, the time of the day, the quality and the quantity of the food taken. Thus, some foods recommended for cold and rainy weathers are strongly inadvisable during summer; a drink that is safe for a healthy individual carries the risk of complicating an already morbid condition, etc. Note was taken too of the accidents connected with prolonged or excessive consumption of some food plants such as the common grass-pea (*Lathyrus sativus* L.) responsible for lathyrism, a disease characterised in the acute state by dorso-lumbar pains, cramps and paresthesia developing into spastic paraplegia.

Rice is the staple food, provided it is of good quality. For example, red rice which grows in marshy areas is considered to be unhealthy. The region of production of cultivated plants therefore has a great importance, as well as the method of cultivation. Wheat ensures good growth and is thought to eliminate the three *doṣa*s. Vegetables must be chosen tender and fresh. Among the most appreciated, we note especially Cucurbitaceae: gourd, cucumber, *Momordica dioica* Roxb. ex Willd., *Trichosanthes dioica* Roxb., *Momordica charantia* L., etc. According to the *Hārītasaṃhitā*, gourd should be known as being of three kinds: small, medium and large [*supérieure*]. Small, it destroys "wind" and stimulates appetite. Medium, it can eliminate the three *doṣa*s. Large, it suppresses swellings, "wind" and "phlegm" and removes "blood-bile. Cooked, it can calm the "bile", it inflames "digestive fire" and cleanses the bladder. Cucumber is constipative and a producer of "phlegm". The leaf of *Trichosanthes dioica* destroys "bile". It is also said that its stalk destroys "phlegm" and that its fruit calms the three *doṣa*s and can be salutary to one who has fever. The fruit of *Momordica charantia*, acrid and sweet, is a producer of "wind" and "phlegm" when it is green. The texts also mention the pumpkin, many kinds of tuber, Liliaceae (onion and garlic), and several chenopodiaceae. Of all the plants consumed as vegetables, the tuber of *Amorphophallus campanulatus* Blume is said to be the best.

Among the fruits, the pomegranate, the myrobalan, the raisin, the date and the lemon are particularly recommended. The fruits of several other plants are also mentioned. The fruit of *Grewia asiatica* L., for example, is especially recommended against disorders of the "wind" and "bile".

Meat also has its place in food prescriptions. According to the *Hārītasaṃhitā* (Prathamasthāna, XXIII, 23), "there is nothing else that is equal to meat to ensure the growth of the body", and the flesh of carnivorous animals is considered as superior because it is packed with meat. But the flesh of animals which have died of old age, or which are lean, or too fat, or too young, that of the animals killed by poisoned arrows or bitten by snakes is reputed to be unhealthy. It is to be noted in this regard that, contrary to a belief widely prevalent in the West, Indians are not a vegetarian people. As regards those among them who are vegetarian, they are so by religious conviction and not with a prophylactic end in view. Even among this category the consumption of meat is allowed when the state of health requires it: "He commits no sin who eats meat when it is consecrated and when it serves as a cure" proclaims the *Mārkaṇḍeya-Purāṇa* (XXXII, 20). Other texts authorise the consumption of meat without consecration or restriction in case of famine or sickness. Even when blood is prescribed by the physician he commits no sin because it is the application of a rule.

Vegetable oils and fatty substances of animal origin have a number of uses, as much in cooking as in therapy. The same is true for sugarcane products (*Saccharum officinarum* L.) and spices.

Milk and milk products occupy an important place in food and health prescriptions. Milk is generally considered to purify the organic vessels and calm the three *doṣa*s. The medical texts inform us also about the properties of yoghurt, which vary from one season to the other. In spring (March-May), in summer (May-July) and in autumn (September-November) yoghurt is not of good quality. By contrast, during the rainy season (July-September), in winter (November-January) and during the cold season (January-March) it is reputed to be salutary. Nevertheless, it is not advisable to those who suffer from diseases accompanied by bleeding, skin diseases, icterus, consumption or acute rhinitis. Buttermilk, butter, and the froth of milk also have very precise indications and counter-indications. Fresh butter, for example, is considered as an excellent stimulant of "digestive fire".

Water is the drink *par excellence*, provided that it is pure. Polluted water and waters in which worms and insects abound are unfit for consumption. It is likewise inadvisable to bathe in them for they can cause itching and skin eruptions. The properties of potable water depend on its provenance. Popular literature proclaims the beneficial and purificatory virtues of the water of sacred rivers. According to the *Hārītasaṃhitā* (Prathamasthāna, VII, 103-105), water is preferably to be consumed during the middle of a meal. It then contributes to maintaining the balance of the organic constituents, the *dhātu*s, and facilitates digestion.

Alcoholic drinks also have their place in diet. The *Carakasaṃhitā* lists 84 kinds. Some are studied in detail in the *Suśrutasaṃhitā* which indicates their qualities and defects. In small doses, they are generally considered as tonics, sharpening the appetite, facilitating digestion and even eliminating a certain number of diseases, especially the diseases of "phlegm".

The preparation of foods (cooking, seasoning, etc.) and the composition of menus also attract special rules. There is even a *Sūpaśāstra* (Treatise on soups) some extracts of which have passed into medical literature. Ayurveda also speaks of what each person should or should not do before and after a meal. For example, it is inadvisable to take food when one is tired or after much exertion. He who has just eaten must avoid exertion, sexual relations, running, drinking and singing. He should on the contrary take rest, taking a nap. Sleep during the day is moreover advised for sick people, the aged, children, and to those who stay awake during nights.

IV. Tonics and Aphrodisiacs

Various speculations have contributed to accentuating among Indians the natural human tendency ardently to seek the preservation of youth and life. The ancient *vedic* hymns whose purpose was to obtain health and long life are legion. The god Rudra is beseeched for a life of a hundred years. Varuṇa, who in later classical literature became the rain god, is invoked as the guardian of the "liquor of immortality", the *amṛta*, which is manipulated during sacrifices under the name of *Soma*, a plant with wonderful powers and to which the 120 hymns that comprise Book IX of the *Ṛgveda* are wholly devoted. Several authors, since the late nineteenth century, have sought to identify this plant, while others have agreed that *Soma* was quite possibly nothing but a mythological concept. The most appealing hypothesis is that advanced some years ago by an ethnomycologist, R. Gordon Wasson. According to this author, the *Soma* used originally by the Āryans was a hallucinogenic mushroom, the *Amanita muscaria.*[5] What the Brahmins sought to obtain by their ritual and their formulas, and others by magic or by the practice of yoga, the physicians sought from tonics and stimulants, the *rasāyana*s, and from aphrodisiacs, the *vājīkaraṇa*s.

The *vājīkaraṇa*s are believed to increase the strength of those who are weakened and whose virility is low. These are most often preparations based on sesame, broad beans (*Phaseolus radiatus* L.), sweet potatoes (*Ipomea digitata* L.), sugarcane juice, long pepper (*Piper longum* L.), emblic myrobalan and milk, in combination with the testicles of goats, buffaloes or donkeys. The roots, bark, buds and fruits of the *aśvattha* tree (*Ficus religiosa* L.) are also used.

As regards the *rasāyanas*, they are elixirs which are expected to confer long life, health and youth. The *Carakasaṃhitā* gives very detailed instructions for their preparation. One of the most famous is the *Cyavanaprāśa* in the compounding of which more than 30 ingredients figure. Among the major drugs used in the preparation of these "elixirs of long life" figure the following plants: *Zizyphus napeca* Willd., *Terminalia tomentosa* W. & A., *Carpopogon pruriens* Roxb., *Phaseolus trilobus* Ait., *Teramnus labialis* Spreng., *Gymnema aurantiacum* Wall., *Tinospora cordifolia* Miers., *Rhus succedania* L., *Prunus puddum* Roxb., *Hydrocotile asiatica* L. Caraka prescribes the last-mentioned plant as an ingredient in the preparation of the *Aindra Rasāyana*, an elixir of health recommended in cases of chronic diseases, which is also believed to increase memory and intelligence. It is also prescribed in preparations against mental disorders. According to the *Rājanighaṇṭu*, a Sanskrit dictionary of the thirteenth century, the *Hydrocotyle* "is cold, astringent and bitter. It eliminates wind and diseases that result in bleeding. It can produce the awakening of consciousness, comprehension and intelligence; it increases vitality". Hence it is considered above all as a neurotonic and a general stimulant. The *Hydrocotyle asiatica* has long been known in Europe where it has been used against insanity and epilepsy, in conformity with Indian usage. It has also been tried against leprosy by virtue of its vulnerary effects. In case of fever, it is an effective diuretic, which soothes the heart and causes a lot of water to be eliminated. This action is essentially due to a triterpenoid saponin: *asiaticoside.*

For their part, the tantric schools of haṭhayoga developed sexual practices comparable to those of Chinese Taoism and in which coitus appears, not as an act meant for procreation or for satisfaction of the libido, but as a means of acquiring, if not immortality, at least a state of superhealth. It was thought that this state could be reached by avoiding during sexual intercourse any emission of sperm or by reabsorbing it. The technique taught by the haṭhayoga consists in compressing the urethra at the moment of ejaculation. It implies also a phenomenon of vesicular aspiration by the action of the muscles of the abdominal wall, as in the case of internal enema (*basti*) already mentioned.

V. The Preventive Application of Massages

Massages as they are practised today, especially in south India, are mentioned in the oldest Sanskrit medical texts which cite their different techniques with their major indications and counter-indications. There is special mention of these in the chapters of these books which treat the rules to be observed daily to remain in good health. Indeed, āyurvedic massages not only constitute a form of therapy, but are also, with general hygiene and diet, a means of prevention. That is why they are recommended to healthy individuals with the aim of relaxation.

There are several types of āyurvedic massage which are done with bare hands, with or without oil, and sometimes even with the feet. These different techniques (effleurage, rubbing, pressing, kneading, pinching, tapotement, rolling) can be combined with each other and may be combined with plant poultices as well as with *pañcakarman* therapy (see chapter IV, I).

The Sanskrit texts do not content themselves with mentioning these techniques and their indications, they also specify the conditions under which these different massages can and should be done. These conditions concern the type of patient on whom the masseur should operate, their sex, their age, their temperament, their state of health. The indications and counter-indications are also a function of the climatic conditions, the time of the day, etc. In general, a massage is indicated in the prevention of diseases attributed to an excitation of the "wind" or of the "phlegm". That is why sesame oil massages are recommended during the rainy season when the "wind" and the "phlegm" are the most excited. Sesame oil penetrates the tissues very quickly and warms them up. According to the *Carakasaṃhitā* (Sūtrasthāna, V, 85-86) oil massage strengthens the body, makes the skin smooth and prevents disorders of the "wind".

Oil massages of the head and the feet have the effect of removing fatigue and inducing sleep. Coconut oil is generally used for the head. The *Suśrutasaṃhitā* specifically forbids body massage in case of indigestion, high fever or for a patient being treated by emetics and purgatives. Aside from that, massage is recommended after a bath. All the muscles must be massaged, kneaded one by one, and the scalp must be rubbed with oily preparations.

A common practice in south India is the "oil bath" which consists in smearing oil on the body from head to foot several times a week. The body is massaged, then it is rubbed with an absorbent paste to remove the excess oil before being sprayed with hot water or taking bath. The oil bath is particularly recommended for babies and young children.

Notes

1. J. Filliozat, Sur la concentration oculaire dans le yoga, *Zeitschrift Yoga*, 1, 1931, pp. 93-102.

2. Also known as *paścimottānāsana*.

3. Th. Brosse, *Etudes instrumentales des techniques du yoga*, preceded by *La nature du yoga dans sa tradition*, by J. Filliozat, Paris, Ecole française d'Extreme-Orient, 1963.

4. See G. Mazars, La diététique âyurvédique, Proceedings of the Symposium *Alimentation et médecine,* Brusssels, Archives et Bibliothèques de Belgique, pp. 11-28.

5. R.G. Wasson, *Soma, Divine Mushroom of Immortality*, new edition, New York, Harcourt, Brace, Jovanovich, 1971. See also, by the same author, The Soma of the Rig Veda: What was it?, *Journal of the American Oriental Society*, 91, 1971, pp. 169-87; Qu'était le Soma des Aryens? in P.T. Furst, *La chair des Dieux*, Paris, Editions du Seuil, 1974, pp. 204-18.

CHAPTER 4

THERAPEUTIC METHODS

The choice of a therapy depends not only on the disease diagnosed but also on the causes which are attributed to it in relation to the excessive activity or improper functioning of the three vital principles (wind, bile and phlegm), the temperament and the environment of the patient. Ayurvedic treatments are therefore individualised and, given the role attributed to faults in behaviour and to dietary lapses in the production of diseases, they give great importance to prescriptions of diet and hygiene.

I. The *"Pañcakarman"* Therapy

The *pañcakarman* therapy is considered as the method of treatment *par excellence* for restoring the normal balance of the three vital principles. Under this name are grouped "five procedures" (*pañcakarman*): the administration of emetics (*vamana*), purgatives (*virecana*), enemas (*basti*), errhines (*nāsya*), and bloodletting (*raktamokṣana*). The months of July and August constitute the best period for this type of treatment. Its duration can vary from seven to fifteen days in most cases.

The administration of emetics consists in orally evacuating the *doṣa*s in excess by prescribing emetics. Among the most usual is the fruit of *Randia dumetorum* Lam. Emetics are prescribed in cases of ailments attributed to disorders of the "phlegm". They are counter-indicated in the case of consumptive disease, in case of weakness, for children, for the aged and for pregnant women.

Purgatives are administered for eliminating by the lower tract the impurities accumulated in the intestines. Castor oil combined with various plants is the most frequently used purgative. Purging is indicated in the case of diseases that result from an imbalance of the "bile": fever, skin disease, digestive disorders, urinary disorders, eye diseases, etc. And it is counter-indicated for children and old people, as well as for pregnant women.

Enemas are intended to purify the organism. The process owes its name to the bladder (*basti*) used for introducing various medicinal preparations into the body. The old texts already distinguish several types of rectal and vaginal enemas, depending on the affections to be treated and the nature of the substances to be injected. Rectal injections are especially indicated in case of fever, diarrhoea, constipation, colic and flatulence.

Āyurveda recommends taking medicinal preparations through the nose (*nāsya*) to rid the head and the neck of the affections which are located there, or, in other words, besides headaches and articular pains of the neck, oral affections and the diseases of the ear, throat and nose. The old medical texts already distinguish some twenty types of such diseases. The prescriptions are powders and nasal drops whose choice, time of administration and dosage depend both on the affection diagnosed and the vital principle (wind, bile or phlegm) involved in the production of the affection.

As regards bloodletting, it is for ridding the organism of "polluted" blood and for combating in this way various diseases for which blood is thought to be the seat, or the source, in particular the diseases of the skin. Anemia, pregnancy, fatigue and old age constitute the major counter-indications. Bloodletting can be carried out by means of lancets or by the application of leeches. Winter is considered to be the best period for bloodletting. In summer, it can be done in the morning or in the evening.

Besides these five "principal measures" (*pradhānakarman*) the *pañcakarman* therapy also includes preliminary measures (*pūrvakarman*) and aftercare measures (*paścātkarman*). The preparatory measures are oleation (*snehana*) and sudorification or inducing sweating (*svedana*). Oleation is believed to destroy "wind" that has become abnormal and to eliminate the impurities obstructing the body canals. It consists in the administration of fatty substances (vegetable oils, animal fats) internally and externally, during several days, in doses and according to frequencies which can vary from one individual to another as a function of various criteria: season, age, temperament and state of health of the patient, and therapeutic indications. Sudorification, ranked among the preliminary measures of the *pañcakarman* therapy, is sometimes one of its major ones or is practised in aftercare. It includes different processes intended to provoke a localised or generalised sweating with a therapeutic purpose. One of the most in vogue, called *piṇḍasveda*, is a massage of the body, or only a part of the body, previously anointed with oil, with balls of a hot paste tightly wrapped by a cotton cloth. Another technique of *svedana* consists in making the patient stretch himself on heated stones covered by leaves. The body can also be splashed with very hot decoctions. In all the cases, the body of the patient must be coated with oil or fat. After each session, the body of the patient must be rubbed down, massaged and the body must take a hot bath.

This kind of physiotherapy is most fully developed in the south of India where therapists are specialised in massages using the feet for treating osteo-muscular lesions. In Kerala, traumas and rheumatic affections are treated by massages and manipulations. Certain methods necessitate the combined skill of several practitioners. In the *pizhichil* technique, for example, the body of the patient is stretched on a special table. Two practitioners are stationed on each side of the upper limbs and trunk of the patient, two others at the level of the pelvis and lower limbs. With their right hands they squeeze a cloth soaked in a medicinal oil over the patient, while massaging him lightly with the left hand. An assistant gathers up the oil which flows from the massaging table, heats it up and pours it into receptacles in which the cloths are soaked. This type of treatment is indicated for treating rheumatic affections and paralyses.

II. Drugs of Natural Origin

The largest number of drugs recommended by Āyurveda are plant-based. In the course of the centuries, āyurvedic medicine has used more than 3000 plant species of which a good thousand still enter, in various forms, into the composition of the remedies prescribed today. One notes also the use of a certain number of substances of animal or mineral origin. Among the animal products figure foods of animal origin, meats, fats, milks and derivatives, as well as blood, bones, nails and horns. The medical texts speak highly also of the beneficial effects of human urine and that of different animals. Goat's urine, for example, is particularly recommended in cases of cough, breathlessness, icterus, anemia or hemorrhoids. Horse's urine, pungent, caustic and warm, is especially indicated in cases of perturbations of "wind" or of "phlegm". As regards human urine, it has been used in salves for treating certain eye affections. The mineral products of the āyurvedic pharmacopoeia comprise notably quicksilver, bitumen, stibnite, realgar, copper sulphate, gold, silver, lead and iron. The last mentioned was used very early, in the form of powder, in the treatment of anemias. One notes also the use of lye obtained from ashes of plants.

All these natural substances have contributed to the manufacture of thousands of remedies often involving very complex formulas. This complexity of the compositions is explained simultaneously by the āyurvedic pathology, by the complexity of the cases to be treated and by the concern for combining the different ingredients in such a way as to counterbalance, increase or prolong the effects of some by the properties of the others. Other substances figure quite simply in the formulas as flavouring agents or as excipients.

The forms of drug delivery are varied: powders, infusions, decoctions, macerations, electuaries, pills, liniments, ointments? Apart from aqueous preparations, the usual excipient is oil or clarified butter (*ghṛta*), but milk and honey are also used. As regards the methods of administration of these remedies, they depend on the nature of the medicine and/or the location of the disease. A certain number of preparations are administrated orally, through the nose or through the rectum (enemas, suppositories). Others are reserved for external use. These are liniments, ointments, eyewashes, sprays.

1. **The āyurvedic theory of savours :** In order to explain the properties of the different substances and their effects on the organism, Indian physicians of antiquity developed theories which apply as much to food as to plants and to the substances of animal or mineral origin in the pharmacopoeia. For that reason they were very early led to establish correspondences between the vital principles and the simplest perceptible properties of these substances such as their consistency, their odour, their colour and above all their savour.

   According to Āyurveda, there exist six basic "essences" (*rasa*) which give their savours to the substances: sweet, sour, salt, pungent, bitter and astringent. For a long time modern physiology only recognised four of them (sweet, sour, salt and bitter), but no one ever thought of verifying their primary character experimentally. In fact we know today that there is no basic savour.[1] Āyurvedic medicine teaches that substances with a sweet, sour or salt savour calm the "wind" but irritate the "phlegm". On the contrary, those which are pungent, bitter or astringent combat the harmful effects of the "phlegm" but excite the "wind". As regards the activity of the "bile", it is reduced by sweet, bitter or astringent substances and increased by sour, salt or pungent substances. Of the six savours distinguished by Āyurveda, the sweet savour appears as the most important for it has been thought to contribute to long life. But an excess of remedies or foods with sweet savour, by perturbing the "phlegm", provokes obesity, promotes laziness, weakens the power of digestion and leads to all kinds of diseases.

   The complex tastes of most substances are interpreted as combinations of two, three, four, five or all six basic savours. In this way are obtained 15 combinations of two savours, 20 of three, 15 of four, 6 of five and one of six, that is a total of 63 different savours. Finally, there exists an infinite number of savours according to the strength of each of the basic savours in a combination.

2. **"Hot" and "cold" substances :** Observing that foods and remedies do not provoke the effects proclaimed by the theory of savours, the theoreticians of Āyurveda sought other explanations to account for the properties of all the substances. They were thus led to establish for each substance:
   A. its "postdigestive" (*vipāka*, literally "after cooking" [by the "digestive fire"]) effect, which flows from its savour;
   B. its "quality" (*guṇa*);
   C. its "potency" (*vīrya*).

   Finally, to explain the exceptions to these rules, the notion of *prabhāva* or "specific action" was developed. These different conceptions conditioned the methods of choice, recommendation and preparation of foods and the medicines.

   Regarding the "potency", for example, āyurvedic pharmacology takes into consideration the thermal qualities of the foods and the remedies. Thus, medicinal plants are described as "cold" or "hot", depending on the feeling that they provoke when they are taken.

   The *Suśrutasaṃhitā* observes that the plants which procure a feeling of freshness are those whose taste is sweet, bitter or astringent. From the botanical point of view, one finds among them the leguminous plants, the cucumbers and the grains as well as a large number of trees and shrubs with edible fruits.

   "Hot" plants are those which provoke, by contrast, a feeling of heat. They comprise, according to Suśruta, species with pungent, sour or salty taste such as ginger (*Zingiber officinale Roscoe*), black pepper (*Piper nigrum* L.), onion (*Allium cepa* L.), garlic (*Allium sativum* L.), saffron (*Crocus sativus* L.) or white pepper (*Brassica alba* L.).

3. **The classification of medicinal plants :** These conceptions are at the root of the classification of the natural substances suggested by Suśruta in the first part of his treatise. But in another chapter (*Sūtrasthāna*, XXXVIII, 1-37), he classifies them into 37 groups, according to the diseases against which

they are used. In the first group are ranked, for example, those which are believed to remedy the disorders of the "bile" and the "wind" and cure the consumptive diseases, tumours, pains of the limbs or also cough and respiratory difficulties. The most noteworthy among them are the following: *Desmodium gangeticum* Dc., *Ipomea digitata* L., *Sida spinosa* L., *Tribulus terrestris* L., *Uraria picta* Desv., *Asparagus racemousa* Willd., *Ichnocarpus frutescens* R. Br.

In the *Carakasaṃhitā* (Sūtrasthāna, IV, 1-74), medicinal plants are divided into five categories, according to their effects on the organism. There are also listed plants "which prolong life", those which make one put on or lose weight, those that are laxatives, appetisers, analeptics, stimulants, anthelmintics, antidotes, galactagogues, emollients, diaphoretics, emetics, purgatives, those that counteract thirst, those that counteract hiccups, those that counteract coughs, plants that are diuretic, antipyretic, analgesic, etc.

4. **Āyurvedic preparations :** Āyurvedic preparations are grouped under four major categories: extracts (*kaṣāya*), preparations based on fatty substances, products of fermentation, and a fourth category which groups all other types of preparations. Included among the "extracts" are: saps and juices of fresh plants (*svarasa*), powders and pastes (*kalka*), decoctions (*kvātha*), macerations (*hima*), infusions (*phāṇṭa*). The second category of preparations comprise remedies prepared with vegetable oils or animal fats into which various mixtures of plants are put to cook. As regards fermented preparations, they are of two kinds. Some, called *āsava*, are obtained by leaving medicinal plants to ferment in water. Others, called *ariṣṭa*, are obtained by the fermentation of decoctions. The last category of preparations groups confections (*avaleha*), pills (*guṭikā*), syrups (*pānaka*) and alkalis (*kṣāra*), among others. Before being administered or incorporated into a mixture, some ingredients, notably toxic plants such as aconite, must be subjected to a special processing or *śodhana* (literally "purification") intended to reduce or eliminate their undesirable effects.

a) Powders : The powders used in āyurvedic medicine

are often mixtures of several ingredients of plant origin (leaves, roots, barks, fruits à), dried, finely powdered and sifted, to which mineral or animal substances are sometimes added. These mixtures can be used directly as an external application (on wounds, ulcers, etc.) or administered orally. They serve also in the preparation of other remedies: decoctions, pastes, etc. The plant powders reserved for external use (powder for massages, for example) are mixed with clay and other components of mineral (zinc, sulphur) and animal (milk) origin.

b) Infusions, decoctions, macerations : There exist several ways of preparing infusions, decoctions and macerations, depending on the type of disease to be treated and the effect desired.

Decoctions, for example, are prepared with dried ingredients that are more or less finely divided, or with powders. For one part of ingredients four parts of water are used. The mixture must be reduced to one quarter on slow fire, by stirring frequently, then cooled and filtered. Often, the process is actually longer. After reduction to one quarter, one can again add four parts of water and continue to heat until reduction afresh to a quarter. The same process may be repeated several times before cooling and filtration. In this way, a very concentrated aqueous solution is obtained. Such decoctions are used in dermatology and for the treatment of wounds.

c) Medicinal oils and butters : Medicinal oils and butters are prepared according to similar procedures. Indeed, for these two types of preparations essentially three kinds of components are used:

1) a liquid preparation, which can itself be a mixture, and consist of decoction(s), fresh extract(s) of plant(s), etc.;

2) one or several ingredient(s) in the form of powder;

3) an oil or clarified butter (*ghṛta*).

In general, if the recipe does not indicate any particular proportions to be observed, the mixture is constituted by one part of the powder(s) to four parts of oil or clarified butter and sixteen parts of liquid preparation. There are some exceptions:

i) When no special liquid preparation is specified, the mixture is made up of one part of powder(s) to four parts of oii or clarified butter and sixteen parts of water or a liquid preparation.

ii) When the liquid preparation consists of decoction(s) or fresh sap(s) of plant(s), a sixth part of powder and an eighth part of oil or clarified butter should be added.

iii) When the recipe includes four or fewer aqueous preparations, each is to be added in a quantity that equals four times the weight of the oil or of clarified butter.

iv) When the recipe includes more than four aqueous preparations, the quantity of each must be equal to the weight of the oil or clarified butter.

v) When the recipe does not include a powder, it is replaced by an equal amount of aqueous extract.

Powder(s) and decoction(s) and/or juice(s) are well mixed. Oil or clarified butter is then added and the mixture is heated. It is stirred regularly to prevent the powder from sticking to the bottom of the receptacle, until all the water evaporates. At the beginning and towards the end, heating on very slow fire is recommended, and the operatrion may last from one to five days according to the nature of the ingredients and the quantities used. In India, the consistency of the medicinal oils and butters can be solid, soft or liquid depending on the room temperature.

d) Pastes and pomades : Pastes and pomades are generally prepared with powders mixed with a liquid, which may be water, cow's urine, a vegetable oil or clarified butter, until the desired consistency is obtained. These preparations cannot be preserved for longer than three or four weeks.

III. Surgical Treatments

Today limited to minor operations, such as bone setting and to reductions of dislocations and fractures, āyurvedic surgery was once probably the most remarkable in Euro-Asiatic antiquity.

The *Suśrutasaṃhitā* mentions 8 operating techniques (incision, excision, scarification, puncturing, catheterisation, extraction, draining and stitching of wounds) as well as 121 instruments and accessories divided into two categories. The first comprises "cruciform" instruments, pliers, bone and dental forceps, speculums, catheters and various accessories, notably operating tables and sloping beds for fractures. The second category groups the cutting instruments: scalpels, saws, scissors, lancets, needles of all kinds and trocars. Several varieties of dressings and bandages were used and haemostasis (arrest of bleeding) was practised by searing with burning heat or chemical cauterisation (application of astringent preparations or ashes), compression, vascular section and the ligature of vessels.

The *Suśrutasaṃhitā* also describes surgical operations which reveal the great daring of the surgeons of that period: the lowering of cataracts with a needle, grafts for repairing the nose and the earlobe, perineal lithotomy for extracting vesical calculi, resection of scrotal elephantiasis, caesarean section, surgical removal of a dead foetus from the womb.

The *Carakasaṃhitā* and the *Suśrutasaṃhitā* even teach a very daring procedure for intestinal sutures which avoids the use of non-absorbable threads whose intolerance by the tissues had been recognised. This procedure consists in bringing the edges of the wound together and having them bitten by black ants. The bodies of the ants are then cut off from the head, whose mandibles serve as staples. It only remains thereafter to close up the abdomen by ordinary suture:

"In case of intestinal occlusion and abdominal effusion, first make the patient sweat, then anoint him with creamy or unctuous substances; then make an incision in the abdomen to a length equal to four fingers, below the navel, and at a distance equal to four fingers to the left of the hairline; then extract the intestines, examine them attentively, and remove the stone creating the obstacle in the intestine of the patient affected by intestinal occlusion or concretion or the obstacle which results from the waste products; then anoint the intestines with honey and clarified butter and arrange them in place as they were before: suture the external wound of the abdomen. In case of leakage due to perforation, first extract the tip of the arrow, then evacuate the intestinal discharge, then adjust the perforated intestine, then make black ants bite it. After the bite, remove their bodies leaving the heads, then suture as before. The bringing together of the edges of the cutaneous wound must be done as described, then an anointing of black earth mixed with liquorice should be applied, then a bandage should be applied as treatment. Then, after having brought the operated patient to a quiet place, aftercare must be prescribed, and he must be installed in a vat of oil or clarified butter while putting him on a milk diet" (*Suśrutasaṃhitā*, Cikitsāsthāna, XIV, 20-21).

This was the procedure in case of laporotomy for penetrating wounds of the abdomen and for intestinal occlusion. But instances of success must surely have been rare. One of the commentators on the passage quoted above observes moreover that the outcome of the operation was very uncertain. That was no doubt why the method is no longer taught in the later treatises. It was however resumed by the Arabs and it was still used, in the first half of the twentieth century, on the Somali coast where the French adventurer Henry de Monfreid (1879-1974) was witness to an operation identical to that described by Suśruta as reported by him in his book *Les secrets de la mer Rouge* (Secrets of the Red Sea) (1932).

Today, āyurvedic orthopaedists are specialised in the treatment of sprains and fractures. They proceed by manipulation, applications of oil and massages. Fractures are treated not by immobilisation by plastering but by bandages preceded by the application of oil and by massages.

IV. Psychiatric Treatments

The psychiatric treatments recommended by Āyurveda scarcely

differ, in their principles, from the treatments recommended for other diseases. They also aim to reestablish the normal balance of the somatic *doṣa*s ("wind", "bile" and "phlegm") as well as the psychic *doṣa*s (*rajas* and *tamas*).

The *pañcakarman* therapy is very much used, notably the procedures *vamana* and *snehana* mentioned above. In particular, the administration of fatty substances (*snehana*) internally and externally is believed to destroy the "wind" held responsible for motor and mental disorders. Application of medicinal oils on the head is also recommended.

All kinds of plant-based remedies are also prescribed among which we find the following species: *Acorus calamus* L., *Bacopa monnieri* Pennel, *Nardostachys jatamansi* DC., *Rauwolfia serpentina* Benth., *Sida cordifolia* L. *Bacopa monnieri* Pennel, for example, is anxiolytic and psychostimulant. It has been used in āyurvedic medicine to improve memory and fight stress resulting from lack of sleep. *Sida cordifolia*, which is a stimulant, has the reputation of controlling the "wind".

Āyurvedic medicine proposes also a form of psychotherapy based on spirituality: cultivating serenity, entertaining spiritual thoughts, reciting sacred formulas (*mantra*) or else going to the temple.

V. Chemical Therapy

It is above all Siddha medicine which has made the most extensive use of remedies derived from natural mineral substances, or after they have been subjected to more or less complicated chemical treatments.

Many of these medicines are still used. Prepared today in special laboratories, they can offer guarantees of dosage and constancy in action.

In several Tamil medical texts, medicinal substances are divided into two categories: the "male" substances and the "female" substances, manifestly by virtue of their combining properties. To the male substances correspond 25 salts or products considered as "salty" including salt, saltpeter, potassium nitrate, alum, borax, camphor and ambergris. Twenty-two other products comprising metals are considered to be similar to them. Mica, iron, mercury, gold, lead, orpiment and talc are notable. To the female substances correspond 4 acids and 22 other substances considered to be like acids, including the oil of *Asclepias gigantea* R. Br., vinegar, sour mango, copper sulphate and sorrel. But this classification, based in practice on savour, is not very rigorous, for certain substances are ranked sometimes among the "salts" and sometimes among the "acids". It differs furthermore from that which is encountered in the Sanskrit texts of medical chemistry and alchemy in which the bodies are categorised into *mahārasa* or "great essences", *uparasa* or "secondary essences", metals, gems and poisons. Among the *mahārasa* are ranked cinnabar, mica, pyrite, chalcopyrite, bitumen, copper sulphate, calamine and a compound of bismuth. The *uparasa* comprise red ochre, iron sulphate, alum, orrpiment, realgar, antimony and an ore which is probably cassiterite. The metals used are gold, silver, copper, iron, lead, tin and zinc. The principal gems mentioned are tourmaline (sometimes classified among the *mahārasa*), amethyst, diamond, emerald, lapis-lazuli, topaz, sapphire and ruby. As regards poisons, they comprise a certain number of plants including several species of Aconite.

The Sanskrit texts profess, moreover, that mercury is the essence *(rasa)* of the other substances, as Śiva is the supreme being of the Universe. And mica corresponds to the feminine energy of Śiva, his *śakti*, traditionally represented in the form of goddess Pārvatī. We can find in these conceptions the śāktic tendency of tantrism which envisages the divine as a bipolar principle, at once male and female. It is symbolised in Indian alchemy by the union of mercury and mica.

For their part, the Tamil medical and alchemy texts accord a major importance to a substance called *muppu* which seems to have played a role similar to that of the "philosopher's stone" among the Western alchemists. It would seem to be a combination of rock salt and two other unidentified substances. One of them, called *antakkal*, could very well have been calcium carbonate. The other, designated by the name *pūnīru*, is considered at once as "male" and "female".

However, chemical therapy does not constitute the only form of treatment. Siddha medicine also knows the use of the medicinal plants of the āyurvedic pharmacopoeia and attaches a real importance to the practice of haṭhayoga. Astrological considerations apply also to the treatments, by virtue of the correspondence established between the universe and the human body whose different parts are placed under specific signs of the zodiac. Furthermore, a certain number of magico-religious practices are encountered which often perpetuate ancient beliefs of the Vedic period.

VI. Diet

Āyurvedic treatments give an important place to diet, in particular when treating affections attributed to a dietary imbalance. Hence we find in Sanskrit therapeutic texts a great number of dietary recommendations and prescriptions for most of the diseases to be treated.

Rice gruel is suitable particularly to those who suffer from diseases accompanied by polyuria or by vesical lithiasis. Barley gruel can be constipative, if it is hot, and facilitate digestion. Mung bean soup thwarts the perturbations of "bile". It is said to be "the best thing for calming down of the fevers" (*Hārītasaṃhitā*, Prathamasthāna, XIII, 3). The soup of brown lentils is sweet, refreshing, it can destroy the most rebellious parasite. That of red lentils is indicated in cases of diarrhoea, for it is constipative.

The tuber of *Amorphophallus campanulatus* Blume is believed to make hemorrhoids, acute pains, tumours and parasites disappear. Among fruits, the pomegranate is indicated for those who suffer from a disease related to the action of "wind". The emblic myrobalan fruit (*Emblica officinalis* Gaertn.) is considered to be antihelmintic. When accompanying spicy food, grapes (*drākṣā*) act on "bile". It is recommended in case of burns, dryness, fainting, fevers. The date, sweet and nourishing, is beneficial in cases of consumptive disease, burning sensations, in disturbances of "wind" or "bile".

Goat's milk is recommended for fever with cough and diarrhoea That of sheep can be salutary for those who are afflicted by diseases of "wind", but it is inadvisable in cases of hemorrhagic disease. The effects can vary according to whether the milk is drunk warm or cooled, taken in the morning, evening or another moment of the day, according also to the nature of the dish consumed at the same time. Yogurt is strongly recommended in cases of hiccups, hemorrhoids or diarrhoea, and must be consumed mixed with water and salted. The froth of milk is recommended for mild fever, diarrhoea or bad digestion.

Food also plays a major role in the treatments of the different affections which Āyurveda ranks among the "diseases of the blood" (see chap. II, V). In such cases dietary regimes which build up strength are prescribed, notably meat regimes. The meat of certain animals are specially recommended. That of wild deer, for example, is particularly indicated in cases of injury, consumption or anemia. Blood itself is considered as a tonic, a remedy for those who suffer from an insufficiency or loss of blood, for ßblood is increased by bloodû (*Carakasaṃhitā*, Śārīrasthāna, VI, 10). In case of severe hemorrhage, it is recommended that the patient consume the blood of goat or of some wild animal (*Carakasaṃhitā*, Cikitsāsthāna, XI, 25). In cases of diarrhoea accompanied by the discharge of blood (*raktātisāra*), the patient is advised to consume the blood of stag or of goat fried in clarified butter (*Carakasaṃhitā*, Cikitsāsthāna, XIX, 74). Blood also enters into the preparation of a tonic drink to be taken following excessive purgative treatments (*Carakasaṃhitā*, Siddhisthāna, VI, 49-50).

Spices, for which India is renowned, and which have a very important role in Indian cuisine, also have their place in āyurvedic therapeutics. Cinnamon (*Cinnamomum zeylanicum* Nees), cardamom (*Elettaria cardamomum* Maton), ginger, nutmeg, varieties of turmeric and different varieties of pepper are cited in the oldest Sanskrit medical texts and they enter into the preparation of a large number of remedies. Their use in food moreover is the natural outcome of their properties which have been recognised in medicine, at a period when Indian culinary art took its inspiration from āyurvedic dietetics.

Spices enter into the composition of various remedies, notably against conditions affecting the digestive system. Long pepper (*Piper longum* L.), common pepper (*Piper nigrum* L.), ginger (*Zingiber officinale* Roscoe), asafoetida (*Ferula narthex* Boiss.), cumin (*Cuminum cyminum* L.) and caraway (*Carum carvi* L.) figure among the ingredients of preparations prescribed in case of indigestion. The first three are also used in the treatment of obesity. Asafoetida is used in case of colic. Long pepper figures moreover in the recipes for the treatment of asthma. The bark of cinnamon is used for its tonic properties.

VII. Popular Practices

The interest accorded to Āyurveda, to Siddha medicine and to unani medicine, whose practice is recognised and made official, must not make us forget the popular notions and medical practices which the ethnologists have undertaken to study. For, popular medicines of India are not just collections of bizarre beliefs and empirical recipes but often constitute very much living entities in a number of cultural groups. In these circles, despite the scientific influence of Āyurveda, most diseases have been attributed to all kinds of supernatural or magical causes. In tribal communities in particular, the anger of local deities, the action of demons, operations of witchcraft or the evil eye are held responsible.[2]

In popular cults a special devotion to a whole series of dubious deities, capable not only of causing suffering and disease but also of putting an end to them, is frequently encountered. The Tharus of Uttar Pradesh, for example, believe in the existence of seven sisters, goddesses or ogresses, whom they hold responsible for several diseases: Śītalā is the goddess of smallpox; Durgā that of cholera; fever is attributed to Jvālā; Kālakā sends intermittent fevers; Hulakā is at the root of vomiting blood; Purvā confers insanity and Pārvatī causes severe headaches. Devotion to Śītalā is encountered also in Punjab and Bengal. Elsewhere, she is worshipped under other names. Mariatala, also known under the name of Mariammai in Tamil country, plays the same role in the beliefs and popular cults of south

India as Śītalā in the communities of north India.

Among the Saoras of Orissa, certain diseases are associated with deities or demons who take possession of the body of the patient. Beliefs of the same kind are encountered among the Mundas and the Oraons of Bihar.

The spirits of the dead, too, can be producers of disease. The Hos of Bihar believe that women who die during childbirth are transformed into evil spirits to whom they attribute the accidents of childbirth. As regards sorcerers, they are believed to be quite capable of unleashing evil forces and of killing from a distance by charms and incantations, or by acting directly by assuming various forms.

Some of these beliefs and practices are encountered not only in tribal communities or in the most disadvantaged strata of the Indian population. They still persist even in urban circles where the tendency to take refuge in ancestral superstitions is still very pronounced, especially when official medicines remain powerless. Scientific medicines and popular medicines are moreover not incompatible with each other. Both are resorted to according to the circumstances. Thus an Indian patient who is not satisfied by the treatment received in an āyurvedic dispensary will resort to a healer, consult an astrologer or participate in a healing ritual. The healers know also the properties of certain medicinal plants which they are able to use correctly in the most common cases where treatment by a physician is not necessary.

Nevertheless, the various popular attitudes in the face of disease and the practices which flow from them are not entirely original. They are often borrowings made from the Indian systems of medicine.[3] Even in the presence of beliefs and practices which would seem peculiar to certain groups, it would be imprudent to assert their originality so long as the entire Sanskrit and vernacular medical literature has not been studied in detail.

VIII. Veterinary Medicine

In India a veterinary therapeutic tradition developed very early and has perpetuated itself up to the present. Modelled on

Āyurveda, this veterinary medicine is known by a whole specialised literature which tells us about the ancient methods of prevention and treatment of animal diseases in India before the advent of modern medicine. Some of these treatments, as yet little known outside India, are still practised at present.

The oldest Sanskrit text of veterinary medicine that has come down to us is a treatise entitled *Aśvāyurvedasiddhānta* "Complete System of Āyurveda of Horses" attributed to a certain Śālihotra. This text is probably prior to the tenth century. We know of a Tibetan version of it which was prepared at the beginning of the eleventh century. It was also translated into Persian in the fourteenth century. Subsequently several treatises on hippology, hippiatry and the Āyurveda of elephants were composed.

In the area of anatomy the knowledge of the ancient Indian veterinarians seems to have been fairly extensive and is more accurate than that concerning the human body. As regards the physiopathological conceptions in the Sanskrit texts of veterinary medicine, they are those of classical Āyurveda. According to these conceptions, the health of an animal, as that of the humans, depends on the normal balance and proper functioning of the three vital principles, the "wind", the "bile" and the "phlegm". The nosology is similar in its broad features to human nosology, but differs from it in details, except with regard, for example, to the diseases common to horses and men.

As in āyurvedic medicine, prevention occupies an important place. It is based on general and dietary hygiene. The texts lay stress on the layout and maintenance of cowsheds and stables, the different sorts of foods with their qualities and their drawbacks, as well as on the dietary rules to be observed. They underline the importance of moderation in food for the domestic animals and enumerate the undesirable consequences of an excess of food. Furthermore, like Āyurveda, the veterinary tradition of India emphasises methods aimed at strengthening the general state of health, notably by the use of tonic and stimulant preparations.

Apart from surgical operations, therapy consists most often in the administration of medicinal preparations by different routes and under different forms: mixtures of powders, decoctions, electuaries, ointments, sternutatories. The texts lay stress quite particularly on the benefits of using medicinal oils and butters in food, in external applications and in enemas.

In the area of hippiatry, we find also various procedures intended to make horses sweat, techniques of cauterisation, bloodletting and several kind of enemas. Procedures of sudorification, 8 in number, are indicated for treating the sicknesses due to "wind" and to "phlegm". The texts of hippiatry distinguish between violent and mild sudorifics. They specify the method of use of each by indicating the most favourable periods for this type of treatment. Cauterisations with red-hot iron are reserved for the treatment of diseases which neither dietary regimes, nor errhines, nor enemas have been able to cure. The sites to be cauterised and the form and the number of the cauterisations vary according to the case to be treated. We are well informed also on the post-operative care and the precautions to be taken in the days that follow the operations. We note also the use of caustics. As far as bloodletting is concerned, the treatises on hippiatry identify the veins to be bled as a function of the cases to be treated. They tell us also about the counter-indications and indicate the food for "reconstituting" the blood and the remedies to be administered if the bloodletting is substantial.

Notes

1. A. Faurion, Naissance et obsolescence du concept de quatre qualités en gustation, *Journal d'agriculture tropicale et de botanique appliquée*, 35, 1988, pp. 21-40.

2. G. Mazars, Souffrance et maladie dans le monde indien, *Histoire culturelle de la maladie*, Toulouse, Editions Privat, 1980, pp. 275-90.

3. See in this regard the article by J. Filliozat, La médecine et la magie des Santals, *Journal asiatique*, 227, 1935, pp. 277-84.

Chapter 5

THE MEDICAL PROFESSION

In ancient and medieval India, āyurvedic medicine was the "official medicine". We are fairly well informed about its practice until the arrival of the Europeans. Sanskrit literature is quite explicit about the medical profession, at least since the beginning of the Christian era. It throws light especially on the composition of the medical establishment, the conditions necessary for the study and practice of medicine, the place of the physician in society, etc.

I. The Medical Establishment

The vedic sources scarcely provide us any information on the practice of medicine and the status of those who practised it. Having regard to the importance accorded to magical therapy, the priest-exorcist was no doubt the physician *par excellence*. But there existed also itinerant physicians belonging to a circle different from that of the bards and the liturgists that the authors of the *Veda* were. That is at least what we understand from a passage from the *Taittirīyasaṃhitā* (VI. 4. 9) which insistently downgrades them and prohibits a brahmin from taking them into their practices.

There are several terms in Sanskrit to denote a physician: *bhiṣaj*, *vaidya*, *cikitsaka*, *upacāraka*. The first of these terms appears to be the oldest attested. In certain hymns of the *Ṛgveda* this word seems rather to denote a bonesetter. Thus, hymn IX. 112. 1 proclaims: "divergent are the occupations of men; the carpenter wants what has been cut (the wood), the *bhiṣaj* what has been fractured". The second term, *vaidya*, has the meaning of "doctor", "learned person", "savant" (from the root *VID*, "to know"). It is the most used. As regards *cikitsaka*, "he who takes care" of the patients, it is our "physician". The word derives from *cikitsā* "therapeutics", a substantive derived from the desiderative form of the root *CIT*, "to think", whose meaning is "to take care". The last term means "he who applies a treatment" (from *upa-CAR*, "to treat").

The texts distinguish several categories of physicians. Some practised independently, others were attached to dispensaries which also employed auxiliary personnel, yet others practised at the court of a king. The latter occupied a high rank in the hierarchy. For the physician of the palace accompanied the king wherever he went and constantly took care of his health. In particular, he had to ensure the safety of the foods served in the royal family. We know, from the *Arthaṣāstra* of Kauṭilya, that physicians, toxicologists and surgeons followed armies during their campaigns. This text contains also the oldest reference relating to a post-mortem examination with a view to finding out the cause of a sudden and suspicious death. It is indicated therein that in case of sudden death, the body of the deceased should be immersed in oil before being examined. There follows a list of signs which enable one to recognise the true cause of death (strangulation, hanging, drowning, beating, poisoning, snake bite) and the manner by which it could have been camouflaged.

Sanskrit sources also tell us of the existence of itinerant quacks working especially for their own benefit. Āyurveda, which was at that time the "official medicine", has had to protect itself from the claims of these charlatans who really seem to have been one of the scourges of the country. Here is how, according to the *Carakasaṃhitā*, true physicians could be recognised:

"Those who are from a noble family, who have received a completely pure teaching, who possess experience, who are skilful, clean, have a steady hand, a disciplined mind, who have all the instruments, are endowed with all the faculties, who know nature and who know what should be done, those are the friends of life, the destroyers of diseases. Yes, those who are such never have any doubt as regards the knowledge of the body, of the formation of the body and the perturbations of nature. Doubts have left them as regards the deep knowledge of the origin, prodromes, symptoms as well as the treatment of diseases that are easy to cure, difficult to cure, that can be improved, or that are incurable. It is they who declare the triple text of Āyurveda [i.e. concerning etiology, symptomatology and therapeutics], with its *rṝsumṝs* and its developments, with its innumerable remedies of the three categories [i.e. those which cure respectively the disorders attributed to "wind", to "bile" and to "phlegm"]. They are experts in the 33 roots and fruits, the 5 salts, the 8 urines, the 8 milks, the 6 latex and bark trees, the category of remedies concerning the five actions like the purgation of the head, etc., the 28 gruels, the 32 powders and pastes, the 600 purgatives, the 500 herbal teas and, as regards hygiene, on food, drink, diet, standing position, walk, sleep, rest, the measures, the substances, the eyewashes, the fumigations, the errhines, the ointments, the washing, the interruption or the non-interruption of evacuations, physical exercise, the examination with healthy sense organs, the treatment and the good manners they are experts in apprehending, retaining, understanding" (*Carakasaṃhitā*, Sūtrasthāna, XXIX, 7).

As regards those who act in the opposite way, the charlatans (*kuvaidya*), they are "the companions of diseases and destroyers of life" severely condemned by Āyurveda :

"Masquerading as physicians, thorns of society, imitating the rule while leaving it aside, they roam the kingdoms thanks to the negligence of the kings. Here is how they are especially recognised: Strutting about in the garb of a physician, they walk the streets in search of work. Once they learn that someone is ill, they rush to the neighbourhood and, within his earshot, they boast of their own quality of physician, they stress that his physician is giving him an inadequate treatment and continually harp on the defects of that physician. They seek to win over the friends of the patient with pleasing manners, insinuations, polite gesture.... They also say that they are interested in very little remuneration. They constantly monitor the therapeutic action when they start treatment, desirous as they are to veil their ignorance by a feigned skilfulness and, incapable of changing the course of the illness, they explain that the patient does not have the means of treatment, does not cooperate, is without character and, when they see he is nearing his end, they attach themselves to another, after having changed their residence. When in the company of ordinary people, they exhibit their incompetence in describing their competence, and exhibit their lack of intelligence by denigrating the intelligence of the intelligent. When they notice a society of educated men they move away from it as travellers from a redoubtable jungle" (*Carakasaṃhitā*, Sūtrasthāna, XXIX, 8-9).

Furthermore, specialists of veterinary medicine have long existed in India for the major animal species. Several of the medical texts which have come down to us are, as we have seen in the preceding chapter, concerned with the treatment of horses and elephants, on the principles derived from āyurvedic medicine. There were also special rules for the treatment to be given to cows. They are found summarised in a chapter of the *Agnipurāṇa*.

II. Medical Education

The available documents also provide a fairly accurate idea of medical education in ancient India. The education of the prospective physician is similar to that of the brahmanical student in its development.

The teaching is mostly based on the study of medical texts which the student must learn by heart, verse by verse, aphorism by aphorism, with all their commentaries. He is helped in his task by the advice and the explanations of the master who discusses the interpretations to be given for the most difficult passages, in the light of his own experience, for clarifying it and by spelling out its content.

This theoretical teaching is completed by a practical training acquired by observing how the master treats his patients, by helping him to prepare the medicines which he prescribes, by learning when and how to use them. The prospective surgeon must practise by applying the different operating techniques (incisions, extractions, sutures) on gourds, hollow stalks or animal carcasses, and acquire in this way a great skill, before being permitted to operate upon his fellow men (*Suśrutasaṃhitā*, Sūtrasthāna, IX).

The texts that we have do not tell us about the duration of medical studies. It is probable that they had to be very long. According to the legend, the famous surgeon Jīvaka studied medicine for seven years at Taxila, in the north-west of India, with the master Ātreya, before being able to practise.

The *Carakasaṃhitā* attests the existence of oral examinations for giving recognition to medical studies. But the practice of medicine remained subject to a formal authorisation of the king.

Buddhism, which has always accorded a great importance to physical health, has contributed importantly to the spread of Āyurveda by encouraging medical studies. We know moreover that Āyurveda was taught in the Buddhist universities, notably at the university of Nalanda which remained the greatest intellectual centre of India until the Muslim invasions of the twelfth century.

Nevertheless, the teachings of Āyurveda continued to be transmitted from masters to disciples, but without major modifications, despite the considerable number of medical collections which were compiled before the arrival of the Europeans and even after, these collections only repeating the substance of the works that had become classic and to which the definitive authority remained attached.

III. Āyurvedic Ethics

The ethics of Āyurveda were formed around the notions which have their roots in *dharma*. This Sanskrit term, derived from the root *DHṚ* "carry, support, keep, hold in trust" has as its primary meaning "norm" and it encompasses public and private behaviour, as well as social relations, to the extent that they express loyalty to a civic and religious norm. To the [western] notion of "law", *dharma* adds those of "custom", of "morals". The term concerns also reality as regulated by natural laws. *Dharma* ascribes each thing to its place, conforming to a cosmic order. *Dharma* is known to us by a whole literature which has been constituted on the fringe of the *Veda* by the necessity of specifying the role of the castes. The oldest texts belong to the category of the *Dharmasūtra* or "Aphorisms on Dharma". Of indeterminate date, these texts treat the rules relating to the castes, to the initiation and the duties of the brahmanical student, of the duties of the head of the household, rules for ascetics and outcastes, dietary prescriptions, theory of torts and expiations, rights and duties of kings. There is also treated in it religious and juridical questions. It is probable that āyurvedic ethics developed also as a reaction against bad physicians or charlatans who dishonoured the profession.

The beginning of medical studies is marked by an initiation ceremony intended to consecrate the bond which would from then on unite the medical student with the master whom he has chosen, with whom he must reside and whom he must serve, like the brahmacārin his *guru*.

The initiation ceremony is completed with a solemn address by the master to his pupil in which are enumerated the duties and the obligations of the physician. The *Carakasaṃhitā* has preserved for us an example which shows the greatest importance attached to ethics.[1] The future physician is indeed strictly obliged to respect the same rules which are found in the *Hippocratic Oath* among the Greeks. He must not carry arms. He must be entirely devoted to his master. He must pray night and day for the welfare of all beings. He must not betray his patients for his advantage and must not profit from his status for abusing the wife of another. He must dress modestly and refrain from strong drinks. He must refuse his treatment to the enemies of the king, to criminals (cf. *Carakasaṃhitā*, Vimānasthāna, VIII, 13).

Suśruta's treatise contains a similar address. After having taken his pupil by the hand and made him turn three times around the sacred fire, as in the wedding ceremony, the master exhorts him to renounce desire, anger, greed, ignorance, pride, the habit of talking about oneself, jealousy, rudeness, calumny, lying, sloth and all impure acts. He should wear the ochre robe and live the life of an ascetic. In all circumstances, he should be attentive to the least desires of his master. He owes assistance to the brahmins, to his elders and to his friends, to the indigent, to ascetics who come to him, as if he they had been his own relatives. But he should not treat hunters and bird-catchers, nor those who have fallen from their caste, etc. (cf. *Suśrutasaṃhitā,* Sūtrasthāna, II, 5).

Incurable people also must be abandoned to their fate. It is in any case what the *Suśrutasaṃhitā* (Sūtrasthāna, XXVIII, 9) advises with regard to incurable wounds. This custom seems to have been very general in ancient India since abandonment by the doctor has passed into a proverb to signify the most complete abandonment. Suśruta moreover cautions the practitioner who might risk treating a case that appears without hope. He incurs public disgrace. But in certain cases, it could be permissible to attempt a treatment "after having first of all refused".[2]

Āyurveda also tackles the questions connected with the end of life. It is not advisable to persevere in prolonging the life of a patient who has reached the end of his life. Furthermore, over the course of the centuries, Indian doctors have been led to conduct therapeutic trials, if only to determine, for example, the effective dosage of a remedy. There is also a legend according to which a queen who wanted to cure the emperor Aśoka (third century BC) of a serious disease had an autopsy performed on an unfortunate man having the same symptoms as he to determine the cause of the disease. This autopsy revealed the presence of a worm in his stomach which only onion could destroy. This vegetable, although very impure from the Buddhist point of view, was given to Aśoka who got well by the elimination of his parasite.

IV. The Physician in Traditional Indian Society

The intrigues of charlatans, the inability of physicians to meet certain situations, and the abuses of certain practitioners from the earliest times, have certainly contributed largely to the bad reputation from which the practitioners of Āyurveda seem to have constantly suffered.

However, the *Suśrutasaṃhitā* tells us that physicians are recruited among the members of the highest castes of Indian society and that they belong to respectable families. Furthermore these must surely have been most often families of physicians. We know, for example, that the celebrated Vāgbhaṭa was himself the son and grandson of physicians. But with the exception of the most famous ones, whom monarchs attracted to their court, *Vaidya*s appear to have been kept out of society. It is true that their obligation to enter into contact with patients of all social conditions rendered them impure in the eyes of their contemporaries. This is no doubt why the *Laws of Manu* (*c.* second century) exclude physicians from ceremonies. In particular, individuals who are in good health should keep themselves at a distance as much from physicians as from patients. This mistrust is explained perhaps also by the fear of contagion. It was thought, as is taught by the *Suśrutasaṃhitā* (Nidānasthāna, V, 32-33), that certain diseases could be transmitted by direct or indirect contact with a patient.

Furthermore, the competence of the practitioners must have been very variable. They were also distrusted for other reasons. For many the physician also personified disease and death, and making fun of him was defying disease and death. In every period, the satirical literature has held the physicians up to ridicule.[3] In this way, physicians are ridiculed in the *Pādatāḍitaka* "The kick", a comical monologue (sixth or seventh century) which takes us to the midst of the society of the lazy men of the town. The attacks appear more severe after the classical period. In particular, in the written works posterior to the Muslim conquest the physicians are often described as ignorant men or crooks appearing under the guise of respectable people but who are the opposite of the ideal type of physician of the *Carakasaṃhitā*.

The satirical writings denounce also the venality and lechery of some physicians. Must one see in this a sign of the decline of Āyurveda for, by eliminating the Pāla dynasty (eighth-twelveth century), by definitively rooting out Buddhism from India and by destroying its remaining cultural centres, the Muslim invaders dealt a severe blow to Āyurveda and to the other sciences of India, as has been testified, as early as the eleventh century, by the Arab scholar Al-Bīrūnī, when he writes that the Indian sciences are no longer cultivated except in areas sheltered from the invaders.

The famous Kṣemendra, poet in the court of king Ananta of Kashmir (eleventh century), is the author of *Kalāvilāsa* "The play of the arts", a poem illustrating the ruses employed by all sorts of individuals for exploiting their fellowmen. In this play we see in succession a false ascetic, courtesans, forgers, bad physicians and charlatans. In another of his compositions entitled *Narmamālā*, the same author proclaims that "all the misfortunes and all the sufferings of the World" come from "all-powerful functionaries, wicked gurus and ignorant physicians" and he adds a little later "it is not the disease that makes people sick, it is the physician".

The practitioners are not spared by the *Hāsyārṇava* "The ocean of Laughter" of Jagadīśvara, a farce in two acts of the twelfth century. The name of the physician portrayed in this play is *Vyādhisindhu* "The ocean of diseases", son of *Āturāntaka* "death of the patient". The character walks with difficulty because of elephantiasis. He coughs and nervously waves his hand to chase the flies attracted by the pus which flows from his wounds. This does not seem to embarrass his patients. The treatments that he inflicts on them are catalogued in a tirade which grotesquely parodies the *Carakasaṃhitā*.

Some centuries later, in his *Kaliviḍambana* "The Derision of the age of Kali" (seventeenth century), Nīlakaṇṭha Dīkṣita also lets us understand that physicians are ignorant men. He explains that the physician does not need to know anything. He need know nothing of diagnostic and therapeutic methods, "the lady of the household will provide him all the information he will need".

V. Modern Day Training of the Traditional Physician

Since the attainment of independence by India in 1947, the central government and the governments of the states of the union, recognising the services rendered by the traditional systems of medicine, have given them a new impetus for development. In order to avoid incompetent or dangerous applications by untrained practitioners, the study and the practice of these systems have been regulated. Collections of manuals have been published and a number of specialised journals have been launched, notably by organisations like the Central Council for Research in Ayurveda and Siddha (CCRAS).

Presently, the practitioners of traditional medicine are trained in colleges and university departments of traditional medicine. In 1985, according to the statistics published by the Indian Ministry of Health, there were 116 university departments or colleges of traditional medicine and 55 institutes, departments and centres of research devoted to these medicines, as well as more than 12,000 dispensaries and 1664 hospitals, and 290,900 practitioners.[4] In April 1999, there were 238 undergraduate colleges of traditional medicine and 54 post graduate colleges devoted to these medicines, as well as 15,749 dispensaries and 2678 hospitals, and 421,664 practitioners These few figures show the importance accorded to the traditional physicians in the health policy of India.[5]

As far as āyurvedic medicine is concerned, for example, three categories of practitioners are authorised to practise: holders of the degree of Bachelor of Ayurvedic Medicine and Surgery (BAMS), doctors in āyurvedic medicine as well as non-degree holders who were practising Āyurveda before the coming into effect of regulations fixing the conditions for practising this medicine.

From 1977-78, a programme for standardisation of the teaching of traditional medicines has been put in place by the Central Council of Indian Medicine, the organisation entrusted with the control of the training and registration of the practitioners of traditional medicine.

In the colleges, the training leading to the degree of "Bachelor of Āyurvedic Medicine and Surgery" is spread over five and a half years. To be admitted, students should have completed their secondary education in science. The organisation of this teaching is placed under the responsibility of the governments of the states. The programme of studies is divided into three courses of eighteen months each, followed by one year of full-time practice in a hospital attached to the college where the training of the future practitioner is continued.

Among the subjects included in the programme are modern anatomy, physiology, clinical pathology, medical botany, semiology and modern methods of investigation, and lastly therapeutics as well as elements of surgery that are specifically āyurvedic. Examinations are held at the end of each year. This training represents a minimum for the practice of traditional medicine. Proper mastery through the acquisition of experience necessitates several years of practice.

The courses are given in English or in the official language of the state in which the teaching establishment is. The knowledge of Sanskrit is often required. It is in any case necessary for the study of the traditional texts. The traditional method of teaching in force in many of the colleges promotes the relations between the master and the pupil according to the "guru-kula" system. The students are in general housed and fed for the duration of their studies.

For those who wish to specialise, some 20 universities offer the possibility of preparing a doctorate in āyurvedic medicine. The most important as well as the oldest are the Banaras Hindu University (BHU) of Varanasi and the Gujarat Ayurved University of Jamnagar. The duration of the studies is three to four years in the course of which the students can develop their knowledge of one of the branches of Āyurveda. There exists also a special course of one year intended for degree holders in modern medicine who wish to become initiated into Āyurveda. For unani medicine, the biggest centres are the *Tibbi College* of the Aligarh Muslim University, the Nizamiah Tibbi College at Hyderabad and the Hamdard University of Delhi to which are affiliated the Tibbi College as well as the Institute for the History of Medicine and Medical Research (IHMMR) with an important library and a museum of the history of medicine.

As regards the practitioners who do not hold a degree and who have been authorised to practise Āyurveda, unani or Siddha medicine, they have been registered under a special schedule and they do not have the same rights as the degree-holding practitioners. For example, they cannot be employed as physicians in the public sector and are not authorised to prepare drugs intended for sale. Operating especially in a rural setting, they are rather called to treat common diseases.

The continuing training of practitioners of traditional medicine is organised by the faculties of traditional medicine or by the professional associations or organisations in the form of postdoctoral studies, seminars and congresses. Thus, beside the All India Ayurvedic Congress, founded in 1907, have been created different institutions. One of the most recent, the National Association of Ayurveda (Rashtriya Ayurveda Mandal) was founded in New Delhi in 1987. Its membership is open to qualified practitioners holding a degree in Āyurveda delivered by an official organisation (college or university department). These professional associations of practitioners of traditional medicine have played an important role in the recent development of traditional medicine. In particular, they have devoted themselves to defining the limits of good practice and to having them respected by their members. They have endeavoured to promote continuing training and have encouraged the development of clinical research. They have also contributed to the rapid development of a medical press specialised in the area of traditional medicine and pharmacy with the support of the pharmaceutical industry.

Notes

1. The principal passages of the medical texts relating to āyurvedic ethics have been grouped together and published with an English translation by G.D. Singhal and D. Sharma Gaur, *Surgical ethics in Āyurveda,* Varanasi, Chowkhamba Sanskrit Series Office, 1963.

2. Cf. J. Filliozat, Le Kumāratantra de Rāvaṇa, *Journal asiatique*, 1935, p. 56.

3. See in particular L. Siegel, How many Vaidyas does it take to change a lightbulb? The Satire of Physicians in Sanskrit Literature, *Bulletin d'études indiennes*, 3, 1985, pp. 167-93.

4. See: *Indian Systems of Medicine and Homoeopathy in India*, Planning and Evaluation Cell, Ministry of Health and Family Welfare, Government of India, 1987.

5. See: Summary of medical care, medical manpower & medical education facilities available under Indian systems of medicine & homoeopathy as on 1.4.1999, *Annual Report 2000-01*, Indian Systems of Medicine & Homoeopathy, Dept. of ISMH, Ministry of Health & Family Welfare, Government of India, 2001.

For further details see : http://indianmedicine.nic.in/html/ismh/annual/annual.htm

CHAPTER 6

INDIAN MEDICINE AND SCIENTIFIC RESEARCH

Research work in Indian medicine has developed and continued in three complementary directions: historical, philolcgical and anthropological studies on the one hand, research in traditional pharmacopoeia on the other, and lastly clinical studies.

I. Research in Indian Medicine

The first people to take an interest in Indian medicine and to translate Sanskrit medical texts were the Persians, the Arabs and the Tibetans. From the seventeenth century, numerous European travellers – merchants, adventurers, scholars and curious men – attracted by India, have had the opportunity of letting us know the results of their observations on indigenous medical practices. But the testimonies and opinions of most of these observers barely merit examination. They did not really know anything of these practices that they came across by chance and of which they saw only the appearance. Furthermore, the Brahmins, who were the depository of medical knowledge, have scarcely been very communicative with Europeans in revealing to them scientific treasures which they hid even from the Hindus of other castes.

It is only towards the late eighteenth century and the early years of the following century that orientalists attracted the attention of the scientific world to the Sanskrit medical literature unfairly neglected until then. Publications of the texts, translations and studies multiplied. In France, the first doctoral thesis devoted to Āyurveda[1] was defended at the faculty of medicine of Strasbourg in 1858. Its author, Dr. G.A. Liétard (1833-1904), was, with P. Cordier (1871-1914), one of the pioneers of āyurvedic studies, which saw a new development under the impetus of the celebrated Indologist Jean Filliozat (1906-82), who too was a physician. In Italy, one of the pioneers of the study of Indian medicine was the great orientalist from Turin, Mario Vallauri (1887-1964), who has left very significant studies on the history and doctrines of Āyurveda. We owe gratitude also to a number of publications to German, British, Dutch and Swiss specialists. Indian medicine has also interested some researchers in Canada and in the United States. For some years, besides the historians and philologists, who explore the scientific traditions of Indian medicine, ethnologists and linguists have been studying its popular forms. Seminars and symposiums have multiplied. It is following one of these symposiums which was held at Groningen (Netherlands) in 1983 that a European Ayurvedic Society[2] was founded in 1983. In France, a Société des études âyurvédiques (Society of Ayurvedic Studies) was created in June 1984, affiliated since 1990 to the European Society of Ethnopharmacology.

Many of the plants of the Indian pharmacopoeia have since long proved their efficacy. In the sixteenth century, the Portuguese scholar Garcia da Orta was one of the first Europeans to study the medicinal plants of India. His book *Coloquios dos simples e drogas e cousas mediçinais da India* published in 1563 is the fruit of a scrupulous and critical survey of the Indian materia medica. For, Garcia da Orta is not inviting us to a travel account dazzled by exoticism but to the discovery of the learning of another civilisation which arouses in him neither derision for what he does not understand, nor wonder or fascination for conceptions and practices that are different. Subsequently, other European scholars have had the opportunity to notice the effects of the plants used by Indian therapists. Nevertheless, it is only at a relatively recent period that the study of these plants by the methods of modern science has been undertaken, as much in India as in Western countries. Among the earliest works, we must recall those devoted to *Rauwolfia serpentina* Benth., the *sarpagandhā* of the Sanskrit medical texts, which led to the discovery of reserpine. Leonhard Rauwolf was the first in Europe (in 1558) to draw attention to the properties of this Apocynaceae, whereas from time immemorial it enjoyed in India the most flattering reputation as an antidote and a sedative. It was only in 1942 that Chopra and his coresearchers were able to prove the existence of a hypotensive effect by the administration of total root extracts of *Rauwolfia* to animals with experimentally-induced hypertension. In 1953, this effect was identified as due to reserpine which had just been isolated. There have also been attempts to justify the ancestral reputation of *Rauwolfia* as an antidote. Two explanations have been suggested in 1976 by Pierre Delaveau: "On the one hand, the subject bitten by a venomous snake is harrowed by the fear of apparently inevitable death. Now, *Rauwolfia* is a powerful sedative. Furthermore, poisoning by cobra venom is accompanied by disorders of blood coagulation (disseminated intravascular coagulation and fibrinolysis) which lead to a rapid death. Now, reserpine, from recent knowledge, is an inhibitor of fibrinolysis."[3]

As regards the clinical experimentation of traditional remedies they are conducted primarily in India and in the neighbouring countries where legislation allows it. In India itself, these clinical studies represent a significant proportion of current research. As most of these remedies have been used for centuries, such research has above all the objective of verifying the truth of the effects which are attributed to them by tradition and, as a function of the ingredients used, trying to explain their mechanism of action. Thus it has been possible to note objectively from the results of biological tests the efficacy of a good number of well-known preparations of āyurvedic, unani and Siddha medicines. But the determination of the active principle by the methods of modern pharmacology runs into difficulty because of the complexity of the remedies. For, most āyurvedic preparations consist of dozens of ingredients. Furthermore, the same preparation can be used for the treatment of very different diseases. It is difficult, in these conditions, to determine the therapeutic indications of each ingredient exactly and to evaluate its possible effects. However, certain plants are more often indicated for the same disease or against diseases manifesting similar symptoms. One can then suppose that these plants do have a relatively specific action which then remains to be confirmed by laboratory studies.

II. Remedies Still in Current Use

Many of the remedies mentioned in ancient Indian medical literature are still prescribed today. Āyurvedic medicine has especially employed, and still uses, compound remedies whose formulas and methods of preparation are very complex, with various modes of extraction and concentration of the medicinal substances with the help of varied solvents (most generally water and oil). These drugs are generally prepared by the traditional practitioners themselves or in the dispensaries. Some preparations are currently produced commercially on a large scale and have even made their appearance in markets outside India.

Thousands of recipes have been enumerated. Their proliferation over the course of centuries can be explained by the long period of development of Āyurveda (several millennia), by the many localities of development, and no doubt also by the lack of efficacy of some of them which led Indian physicians constantly to look for more active ones, while preserving the ancient formulas considered to be efficacious. Many of these drugs are multifunctional because of the number and nature of the components used for their preparation. This is the case with tonic preparations prescribed as a preventive measure and in the treatment of different diseases.

To give an example, a formula for pills against hemorrhoids contains no less than fifteen ingredients of plant origin according to the indications given by the manufacturer: *Balsamodendron mukul* Hook, *Melia azadirachta* L., extracts of *Berberis aristata* DC., *Phyllanthus emblica* L., *Terminalia chebula* Retz., *Terminalia belerica* Roxb., *Arisaema wallichianum*, *Cassia fistula* L., *Bauhinia variegata* L., prepared in the juices and decoctions of *Commelina salicifolia* Roxb., *Mimosa pudica* L., *Acorus calamua* L., *Blumea lacera* DC., *Caesalpinia bonducella* Fleming, *Amorphophallus campanulatus* Blume.

Among the preparations reserved for external use, we may cite a pomade against light and severe sprains, used as much in human medicine as in veterinary medicine. It is prepared with oils extracted from the following plants: *Abrus precatorius* L., *Acorus calamus* L., *Celastrus paniculatus* Willd., *Hyoscyamus niger* L., *Moringa oleifera* Lam., *Nardostachys jatamansi* DC., *Ocimum sanctum* L., *Saussurea lappa* C. B. Clarke, *Vitex negundo* L. To these oils are added extracts of seven other plants: *Anacyclus pyrethrum* DC., *Colchicum luteum* Baker, *Curcuma amada* Roxb., *Gloriosa superba* L., *Litsea sebifera* Pers., *Myrica nagi* Thumb., *Nerium odorum* Sol. All these plants have been studied and their active principles are known. *Nardostachys jatamansi* is often combined with the oil of henbane *(Hyoscyamus niger)* as antineuralgic. *Ocimum sanctum* and *Vitex negundo* are used as vulnerary drugs in external use. In traditional medicine, the rhizome of *Curcuma amada* is applied on contusions and light sprains. The extract of *Colchicum luteum* is used in external applications against pain.

III. The Indian Pharmaceutical Industry

The history of the Indian pharmaceutical industry goes back to the beginning of the twentieth century. As early as 1901 a small enterprise was founded at Calcutta under the name of Bengal Chemical and Pharmaceutical Works. But until its independence in 1947, India remained largely dependent on Great Britain, Germany and France for its drug requirements. It is only from the 1950s that the Indian Union began to equip itself with a modern pharmaceutical industry which has since developed remarkably. It was helped in its efforts by several countries, notably the Soviet Union and the United States. From September 1958, the Soviet Union offered India technical and financial assistance to catch up with the production of synthetic drugs, alkaloids, plant extracts, hormones and, in particular, antibiotics.

In the course of recent years India has become in her turn an exporter of pharmaceutical products mainly to South-east Asia, the Middle East and Africa. Today, the Indian pharmaceutical industry is represented by more than 300 companies or groups which produce antibiotics, vitamins, analgesics and antipyretics, antimalarials, antihistamines, antihelmintics, antidiarrheals, antidiabetics and also raw materials for the pharmaceutical industry.

Beside this modern industry a fairly important activity around traditional drugs has developed and, at present, laboratories produce and also package, according to modern processes, time-honoured preparations which are sold all over India. There exist today hundreds of āyurvedic specialities which can be obtained in dedicated shops or in pharmacies. More than 150 manufacturers share the market. Among the specialities offered tonics, restoratives and hepato-protectors are prominent. Some laboratories also offer a certain number of cosmetic products. Some of these products are exported from India. They are beginning to make their appearance in the United States and in Europe, notably in Germany where several small laboratories produce even toothpastes whose basic ingredient is *Azadirachta indica.*

In India, the production of traditional drugs is subject to the Drugs and Cosmetics Act of 1940 and the Drugs and Cosmetics Rules of 1945 and their more recent amendments in the same way as modern drugs. Since 1964, a licence has been necessary to manufacture a traditional drug. From 1970, the control of licences has been intensified. The number of the licence as well as the composition of the drug must appear on the packaging. Besides, some laboratories have put on the market new āyurvedic drugs better suited to the current demand. But the rules require that the ingredients of these new drugs should appear in the list of medicinal plants whose use is authorised (about 600 species).

This movement has benefited traditional veterinary medicine which has also undergone a revival and one also finds āyurvedic veterinary preparations in the shops. As an example we may cite a stomachic preparation and tonic produced by a firm in Bangalore and whose formula comprises 59 ingredients. It is recommended for the treatment of digestive disorders (anorexia, dyspepsia, constipation) in cattle, sheep, goats, horses and dogs, and the dose prescribed varies according to the size of these animals. Among its major ingredients of plant origin we note the following species: *Aegle marmelos* Corr., *Aquilaria agallocha* Roxb., *Butea monosperma* (Lam.) Kuntze, *Centratherum anthelminticum* Kuntze, *Curcuma longa* L., *Ferula narthex* Boiss., *Moringa oleifera* Lam., *Piper longum* L., *Punica granatum* L., *Terminalia bellerica* Roxb., *Terminalia chebula* Retz., *Tinospora cordifolia* Willd., *Trachyspermum ammi* (L.) Sprague, *Zingiber officinale* Rosc., which āyurvedic medicine, too, prescribes for their appetite stimulating, digestive, stomachic, carminative or else anthelmintic properties.

IV. Exploration and Development of the Traditional Pharmacopoeia

The cataloguing and identification of most of the plants used for the preparation of the remedies described in the ancient medical literature was completed in the 1970s. Simultaneously their chemical study was undertaken. In India, it is the main activity of the Central Drug Research Institute of Lucknow where more than 3000 plant species have already been studied. Several hundreds have been found to be active. For example, a cardiovascular activity can be shown in *Calotropis procera* (Ait.) R. Br., a plant of the family of the Asclepiadaceae which is mentioned a number of times in the oldest Sanskrit medical texts. The traditional medicine of India uses the flowers and leaves of this plant as an application on wounds and against inflammations. They are also included in preparations against jaundice and different diseases which Āyurveda ranks among the "disorders of the blood". Several other species, including *Colchicum luteum* Baker (a Liliaceae), are believed to have an anti-cancerous activity. In other plants, like *Aristolochia bracteata* Retz. (family of the Aristolochiaceae), a spasmolytic activity has been proved. The whole plant is used, and appetite-inducing and digestive virtues are also attributed to it. A paste prepared with the root is used as an external application against the bites and stings of venomous animals. Among the active plants, we may also cite *Melia azedarach* L. (family of the Meliaceae) which, according to āyurvedic tradition, is believed to have a specific action on hemorrhoids.

Even though chemical and pharmacological investigations have multiplied in the course of recent years, we are far from having completed a survey of all the resources of the traditional medicines of India in the matter of medicinal plants, on the one hand because of the wealth of their pharmacopoeia, on the other hand by virtue of the complexity and the difficulties of this research. Thus, for want of information concerning the nature of the plant part used, the time of harvest, the process of transforming the raw drug into the drug used, or else the disease really targeted by the drug, chemists and pharmacologists have often been misled and have lost precious time, the former in isolating substances devoid of interest, the latter in trying in vain to prove ill-defined effects. For what would be the use of identifying the ingredients of ancient remedies if the disease targeted by these remedies is itself not identified clearly? The data collected on therapeutic indications of the medicinal plants of India have often misled the researchers who have not taken into account the etiological and nosological conceptions of Āyurveda nor the evolution of these conceptions in the course of the centuries. For example, the diseases which Āyurveda has ranked among the diseases of the skin are not all skin diseases in the modern medical sense. Furthermore, certain skin diseases have not been considered as such by Āyurveda which classified them under other categories, notably among the "diseases of the blood", as a function of the āyurvedic conceptions relating to blood and its perturbations. These conceptions themselves have undergone variation in course of time, in such a way that the same Sanskrit name for a disease does not always cover the same nosological reality from one century to another. Lastly, certain diseases have never been uniquely identified by ancient āyurvedic medicine which has grouped them with or mistaken them for other diseases. That is why a good many indications noted in Sanskrit literature or communicated by local informants can appear relatively vague to a western researcher only superficially acquainted with Indian medicine.[4] Despite these difficulties, research has made progress. Some years ago studies made on a species of *Coleus* led to the isolation of *forskolin*, a potent diterpene. Another example is that of the banana, *Musa paradisiaca* L., used traditionally in the treatment of ulcers of the stomach. It has been proved that this action is due to the steroidic glycosides that it contains.[5] We could thus multiply the examples which demonstrate that the traditional applications are often validated.

Several Indian laboratories are currently engaged in research on medicinal plants in collaboration with āyurvedic hospitals and dispensaries where remedies prepared with these plants are in daily use. These studies are continued under the aegis of the Central Council for Research in Āyurveda and Siddha (CCRAS) and the Central Council for Research in Unani Medicine (CCRUM). The 30 most studied medicinal plants of India include *Abrus precatorius* L. (Leguminosae), *Azadirachta indica* A. Juss. (Meliaceae), *Bacopa monnieri* Pennel (Scrophulariaceae), *Psoralea corylifolia* L. (Leguminosae), and *Semecarpus anacardium* L. (Anacardiaceae), on which there is growing research. For, given their multiple uses in traditional medicine, there remains the possibility that new uses for these plants will be discovered. Thus, *Bacopa monnieri,* studied in India, in the United States and in Europe, might find applications in the treatment of Alzheimer's disease.

V. The Future of the Traditional Medicines of India

The traditional medicines of India still have a great future before them, judging by their place in the health policy of the Indian Union and the growing interest that they continue to arouse almost everywhere in the world.

For, the state of economic and cultural evolution of India and its neighbouring countries at present makes the use of Āyurveda, Siddha and unānī medicines a necessity.

From another point of view, the opponents of these traditional medicines fear that the official recognition and organisation of āyurvedic and other studies might perpetuate a form of medicine whose value they contest and which, according to them, ought to disappear. Since the nineteenth century, the advocates of Āyurveda have themselves been divided into two tendencies. Some favour a system integrating modern scientific knowledge. Others, opposed to any syncretism, wish to remain faithful to the tradition of the Sanskrit texts. This opposition between the progressives and the orthodox has done a disservice to traditional medicine in the face of its detractors.

In any case, Indian traditional medicine still renders many services and it seems at present difficult to do away with it. Doing so would go against the national interest, for there are very few practitioners of modern medicine outside the big cities. Furthermore, the judicious exploitation of the resources of traditional pharmacopoeia ought to contribute to reducing the financial burden imposed on India by the importation of costly pharmaceutical products. This makes it necessary to properly manage the plant wealth of the Indian subcontinent. As it happens, over the last few years, growing demand coupled with insufficient or irregular production has made it more difficult to find certain plant species, according to the information published by the Indian Ministry of Health. That is why experts meeting in Manali (Himachal Pradesh) in April 1986, having noticed that several plants were becoming rare, recommended their cultivation and a ban on their export. Another meeting of experts, which was held in Guwahati (Assam) in June of the same year, recommended a ban on the export of 14 plants threatened with extinction. Among these plants figure *Kalanchoe pinnata* Pers. and *Rauwolfia serpentina* Benth. Some months later, in December 1986, a commission of experts, meeting at Nainital (Uttar Pradesh), recommended that the Indian Government take measures to discourage the exportation of medicinal plants and to control domestic supplies. In fact, the production of certain plants, abundant not long ago, has quickly become insufficient in several regions of India even to meet domestic demand. Other plants, still common or abundant in some states of India, are rare in other regions. For example *Abrus precatorius* L. would appear to be rare in Uttar Pradesh; *Bacopa monnieri* Pennel would appear to be rare in the regions of the north-east; *Semecarpus anacardium* L. would also appear to be rare in these regions as well as in the central regions of Uttar Pradesh, Bihar and Orissa, and in certain states of the south of India, notably Karnataka and Tamil Nadu. It is no doubt for all these reasons that the Indian Government banned, in 1993, the exportation of wild medicinal plants. In 2000, a *Medicinal Plants Board* was constituted by the Government of India to ensure availability of medicinal plants and coordinate all matters relating to their development and sustainable use. The Board has identified 29 medicinal plants as endangered and, in September 2001, the Board invited offers from cultivators and users for supply and/or purchase of 16 medicinal plants in the form of crude drugs on an annual basis, including for example *Aconitum heterophyllum* Wall. ex Royle, *Bacopa monnieri* Pennel, *Nardostachys jatamansi* DC., *Saussurea lappa* C.B. Clarke, and *Withania somnifera* (L.) Dunal.

In the West, āyurvedic medicine enjoys the public craze for so-called "alternative"[6] medicines, whose success is explained by the shortcomings of modern medicine. As a matter of fact, the media are making a mistake and misleading the public by categorising Āyurveda among the "alternative" medicines and highlighting the innocuousness of its methods. Such a mixture of ideas is bound to discredit Āyurveda which constitutes in reality an allopathy, treating the diseases with remedies that are of a contrary nature, for example the diseases considered as cold by drugs and a diet that induce heat. Also, Indian medicine ought to be clearly distinguished from all the other practices not based on the experience of modern science. The properties attributed to the remedies of āyurvedic herbal medicine have been validated by rigorous research that has appeared in scientific publications. This is not the case with most of the "alternative" therapeutics. But we must also be aware that the study and evaluation of Indian therapies are still in their early stages.

The public interest in Indian medicine, like that for other non-official therapeutics, at least has the merit of encouraging the practitioners of modern medicine to reflect on their own attitudes in the face of the demands or expectations of patients who are increasingly disillusioned by the biomedical sciences that do not provide the answer to their daily suffering. The pharmacologists, for their part, continue to explore the Indian pharmacopoeia in search of natural substances capable of enriching the modern therapeutic arsenal. This also explains the interest manifested by the pharmaceutical industry. Discovering the activities of extracts or possibly original molecules is however not the sole motivation of the researchers. Their work is also a response to the demands of national and international organisations which are concerned with fully promoting the traditional pharmacopoeias and the resources of the countries of the South.[7]

Notes

1. G.A. Liétard, *Essai sur l'histoire de la médecine chez les Indous*, thesis presented at the Faculté de Médecine de Strasbourg, Strasbourg, printed by G. Silbermann, 1858, p. 64.

2. Since 1990, this association has published the *Journal of the European Ayurvedic Society*, and from 2001, *Traditional South Asian Medicine*.

3. P. Delaveau, Les fonds des pharmacopées traditionnelles et l'expérimentation moderne, *Scientia Orientalis*, 1977, 12, p. 11.

4. Thus, several species of plants (*Acacia catechu* Willd., *Brassica campestris* L. var. Sarson Prain, *Eclipta alba* (L.) Hassk., *Saussurea lappa* C.B. Clarke) have as indication the "diseases of the skin" in general. In fact, they are used in the preparation of a very large number of āyurvedic remedies against diseases that manifest themselves in the skin and that have similar symptoms which āyurvedic medicine considers sometimes as one and the same disease. Conversely, the different phases of the same disease, like leprosy, were regarded as many different diseases in the ancient period. As regards psoriasis, its symptoms were confused with those of at least five diseases which manifest in the skin, distinguished by Āyurveda.

5. T. Sevenet, Les Orientations de la recherche en phytothérapie: Pharmacologie, *Encyclopédie des médecines naturelles, Phytothérapie-Aromathérapie*, Paris, Editions Techniques, 1991, B-8-5, pp. 9-10.

6. The reader may consult, on this subject, F. Laplantine and P.-L. Rabeyron, *Les médecines parallèles*, Paris, PUF, 1987 (1st ed.) in the collection. "Que sais-je?" (no. 2395).

7. G. Mazars, F. Mortier, L'ethnopharmacologie en Europe, *Ethnopharmacologie: Sources, Méthodes, Objectifs*, Paris, Editions de l'ORSTOM/Société française d'ethnopharmacologie, 1991, pp. 43-47.

CONCLUSION

Āyurvedic and Siddha medicines are the fruit of long medical observation, speculation and practice, and have exerted a great influence far beyond the frontiers of the Indian world.

The underlying concepts of these medicines relating to health and disease are not devoid of interest. An understanding of all the organic and psychic phenomena which, if not always true, was at least rational.

The examination of the data collected in the earliest Sanskrit medical texts shows that the physicians of ancient India visualised living beings in a way that we might qualify today as systemic. Humans (as well as animals) are considered as an open system according to a concept fairly close to that developed, some decades ago, by Ludwig von Bertalanffy (1901-72), or in other words a system exchanging matter, energy and information continually with its environment.[1] In the Sanskrit texts this system is described both from a structural aspect and from a functional aspect. Āyurvedic medical practice is also marked by systemic thought. Its overall objective is to maintain the normal balance of the vital principles responsible for the proper functioning of the organism or to reestablish this balance when it is disrupted. Thus, Āyurveda appears as a system which gives greater weight to prevention than to treatment by stressing hygiene, food and environment whose decisive role in triggering certain diseases is being discovered today.

These concepts have two important consequences. In the presence of any disease, even a localised one, the practitioner who relies on Āyurveda will first seek to discover the nature of the perturbation of the vital elements. He must thereafter apply a general treatment tailored to the individual and not be content with administering a topical or symptomatic drug. He will therefore have to treat the sick person and not merely the disease from which the patient is suffering.

If the notions of anatomy and physiopathology remained rudimentary, traditional Indian therapeutics, by contrast, is very rich. Beside physical means: massages, fomentations, sudorific procedures..., it has primarily used medicinal plants in the form of very elaborately compounded remedies, whose judicious use continues to give results that cannot be ignored.

In India, traditional medicines continue to render great service everywhere where modern medicine remains insufficiently spread. In the West, at a time when public health policies are called into question and when there is a preference for methods judged more natural, Indian therapies are subject to a growing interest. Whereas modern medical practice has branched out more and more into specialities which in turn require specialists, the āyurvedic approach characteristically considers the individual in his totality, limits recourse to chemical drugs and on the contrary aims to reinforce the natural defences of the organism. All this explains the attraction and the fascination which Indian medicine exercises over a public that is more and more disillusioned by the current tendencies of western medicine. At the same time, it offers anthropologists, psychologists, physicians and pharmacologists a vast and promising field for research.

Notes

1. Ludwig von Bertalanffy, *General System Theory. Foundations, Development, Applications*, New York, Braziller, 1968.

CHRONOLOGY

ANTIQUITY

Indus civilisation	Circa 2500 BC	Existence of a highly developed urban and private hygiene Exchanges with Mesopotamia
"Vedic" period	Circa 15th-11th c. BC	Composition of the *Veda*; earliest medical data
	Circa 11th-6th c. BC	Redaction of the *Brāhmaṇas* and the older *upaniṣads*
Buddha	Circa 6th-5th c. BC	Jīvaka, father of Indian surgery
Nanda dynasty	350-320 BC	Development of Āyurveda Alexander in India 327-325 BC
Maurya dynasty	320-185 BC	Testimonies of the Greeks
Sunga dynasty	185-75 BC	on medicine and veterinary art in India
Kuṣāṇa dynasty	1st-3rd c. AD.	Fixing of the great medical Saṃhitās of Caraka and Suśruta
Gupta dynasty	320-500 AD	Āyurveda is at its peak
Reign of Harṣa	606-647 AD	Vāgbhaṭa (7th c.?) compiles the *Aṣṭāṅgahṛdayasaṃhitā*
Conquest of Sind by Muslims	712 AD	

MEDIEVAL PERIOD

Local kingdoms	8th-12th c. AD	Treatise on etiology by Mādhava (8th c.), therapeutic collections of Vṛnda (9th-10th c.) and of Vaṅgasena (12th c.)
Muslim conquest	12th c. AD	Introduction of Arab medicine
Sultanate of Delhi	13th-16th c. AD	
Khalji dynasty	1290-1320	Śārṅgadhara (13th-14th c.), author of a medical collection Development of Āyurvedic phygmology
Tughluq dynasty	1320-1413	Ḍiyā Muḥammd redacts the *Majmū-e Ḍiyā'ī* (1336). Madanapāla writes a treatise ofāyurvedic materia medica (1374)
Sayyid and Lodi dynasties	1414-1526	

MODERN AND CONTEMPORARY PERIODS

Mughal dynasties	16th-18th c. AD	Golden age of Unānī medicine; Āyurvedic treatise of Bhāvamiśra (16th c.)
British rule	19th-20th c. AD	Spread of western medicine and revival of traditional medicines
Independent India	Since 1947	Recognition of the traditional medicines. Development of pharmacological and clinical research

BIBLIOGRAPHY

1. *Texts, commentaries and translations*

Bhisagratna K.K., An English translation of the *Suśruta samhita* based on the original Sanskrit text, Varanasi, Chaukhamba Sanskrit Series Office, 1963, 3 vol.

Filliozat J., *Yogaśataka*, medical text attributed to Nāgārjuna, Sanskrit and Tibetan texts, French translation with notes and indices, Pondicherry, Institut français d'indologie, 1979.

The Charaka Samhita, with translation in Hindi, Gujarati and English, Jamnagar, Shree Gulabkunverba Ayurvedic Society, 1949, 6 vol.

Hilgenberg L., Kirfel W., Vāgbhaṭa's *Aṣṭāṅgahṛdayasaṃhitā, ein altindisches Lehrbuch der Heilkunde*, aus dem Sanskrit ins Deutsche übertragen mit Einleitung, Anmerkungen und Indices, Leiden, 1941.

Meulenbeld G.J., *The Mādhavanidāna and its chief commentary*, chapters 1-10, Introduction, translation and notes, Leiden, E.J. Brill, 1974.

Murthy, K.R.S., *Śārṅgadhara-saṃhitā (A treatise on Ayurveda)*, by Śārṅgadhara translated into English, Varanasi, Delhi, Chaukhamba Orientalia, 1984 (Jaikrishnadas Ayurveda Series No 58).

Murthy, K.R.S., *Mādhava Nidānam (Roga Viniścaya) of Mādhavakara (A treatise on Āyurveda)*, Text with English Translation, Critical Introduction and Appendices, Varanasi, Delhi, Chaukhamba Orientalia, 1993 (Jaikrishnadas Ayurveda Series No 69).

Raison A., *La Hārītasaṃhitā*, texte médical sanskrit avec un index de nomenclature âyurvédique, Pondichéry, Institut français d'indologie, 1974.

Sharma P.V., *Caraka-Saṃhitā* (Text with English translation), Varanasi, Delhi, Chaukhamba Orientalia, 4 vol., 1981-1994 (Jaikrishnadas Ayurveda Series No 36).

Sharma P.V., *Cakradatta* (Text with English translation), *A Treatise on Principles and Practice of Ayurvedic Medicine*, Varanasi, Delhi, Chaukhamba Orientalia, 1994 (Kashi Ayurveda Series No 2).

Vogel C., *Vāgbhaṭa's Aṣṭāṅgahṛdayasaṃhitā*. The first five chapters of its Tibetan version edited and rendered into English along with the original Sanskrit, Wiesbaden, Kommissionsverlag, Franz Steiner, 1965.

2. *Books and articles*

Bigot A., *La médecine française ā Pondichéry aux XVIIIe et XIXe siècles*, XCI[e] Congrès des Sociétés savantes, t. I, Rennes, 1966, p. 31-46.

Crawford D.G., *A History of Medical Service in India: 1600-1913*, London, 1914, 2 vol.

Dandiya P.C., Vohora S.B., *Research and Development of Indigenous Drugs*, Delhi, Institute of History of Medicine and Medical Research, 1989.

Dash B., *Fundamentals of Ayurvedic Medicine*, Delhi, Bansal & Co. 1978.

Dash B., *Alchemy and Metallic Medicines in Āyurveda*, New Delhi, Concept Publishing Company, 1986.

McDonald D., The Indian Medical Service. A Short Account of its Achievements, 1600-1947, *Proceedings of the Royal Society of Medicine*, no. 49, 1957, p. 13-17.

Filliozat J., La médecine indienne et l'expansion bouddhique en Extrême-Orient, *Journal asiatique*, avril-juin 1934, p. 301-307.

Filliozat J., La médecine de l'Inde, *La Nef*, no. 23, 1965, p. 19-58.

Filliozat J., *The classical Doctrine of Indian medicine. Its origins and its Greek parallels.* Translated from the original in French by Dev Raj Chanana, New Delhi, Munshiram Manoharlal, 1964.

Huard P., Bossy J., Mazars G., *Les médecines de l'Asie*, Paris, Editions du Seuil, 1978.

Iyengar M.A., *Bibliography of Investigated Indian Medicinal Plants (1950-1975)*, Manipal, Kasturba Medical College, 1976.

Jolly J., *Indian Medicine*, Translated from German and Supplemented with notes by C.G. Kashikar with a foreword by Dr. J. Filliozat, Second revised edition, New Delhi, Munshiram Manoharlal, 1977.

Kutumbiah P., The Pulse in Indian Medicine, *Indian Journal of the History of Medicine,* no. 12 (1), 1967, p. 11-21.

Kutumbiah P., *Ancient Indian Medicine*, revised edition, Bombay, Madras, New Delhi, Orient Longman, 1969.

Leslie C., (ed.), *Asian Medical Systems: A Comparative Study*, Berkeley, Los Angeles, London, University of California Press, 1976.

Mazars G., La médecine indienne classique, *Histoire de la médecine, de la pharmacie, de l'art dentaire et de l'art vétérinaire*, t. II, Paris, Sfemps, 1978.

Mazars G., Souffrance et maladie dans le monde indien, *Histoire culturelle de la maladie*, Toulouse, Privat, 1980, p. 275-290.

Mazars G., La médecine dans l'Inde antique, *Encyclopédie des médecines naturelles, Phytothérapie-Aromathérapie*, Paris, Editions Techniques, 1991, A-1, p. 1-10.

Mazars G., La médecine âyurvédique, *Encyclopédie des médecines naturelles, Phytothérapie-Aromathérapie*, Paris, Editions Techniques, 1991, A-4, p. 1-22.

Mazars G., Traditional veterinary medicine in India, *Revue scientifique et technique de l'Office international des épizooties*, vol. 13, no. 2, 1994, p. 443-51.

Meulenbeld G.J. (ed.), *Proceedings of the International Workshop on Priorities in the Study of Indian Medicine*, held at the State University of Groningen, 23-27 October 1983, Groningen, Rijksuniversiteit te Groningen, 1984.

Meulenbeld G.J. and Wujastyk D. (ed.), *Studies on Indian Medical History*, Papers presented at the International Workshop on the Study of Indian Medicine held at the Wellcome Institute for the History of Medicine, 2-4 September 1985, Groningen, Egbert Forsten, 1987.

Mitra J., *History of Indian Medicine from pre-Mauryan to Kuṣāṇa Period*, Varanasi, Jyotirālok Prakashan, 1974.

Mukhopadhyaya G., *History of Indian Medicine*, containing Notices, Biographical and Bibliographical, of the Ayurvedic Physicians and their Works on Medicine, from the Earliest Ages to the Present Time, Calcutta, University of Calcutta, 1922-29. Second edition, 3 vol., Oriental Books Reprint Corporation, New Delhi, 1974.

Ojha D. and Kumar A., *Panchakarma-therapy in Āyurveda*, Varanasi, Chaukhamba Amarabharati Prakashan, 1978.

Ray P., Gupta S.N., *Caraka Saṃhitā (A Scientific Synopsis)*, New Delhi, National Institute of Sciences of India, 1965.

Rosu A., *Les conceptions psychologiques dans les textes médicaux indiens*, Paris, Institut de civilisation indienne, 1978.

Rosu A. (ed.), *Un demi-siècle de recherches âyurvédiques, Gustave Liétard et Palmyr Cordier, Travaux sur l'histoire de la médecine indienne*, documents réunis et présentés par Arion Rosu, Paris, Institut de civilisation indienne, 1989.

Sharma D.P., Shastri S.K. (ed.), *Basic Principles of Āyurved*, Patna, Shree Baidyanath Ayurved Bhawan Ltd, 1978.

Sharma P.V., *Indian medicine in the classical age*, Varanasi, Chowkhamba Sanskrit Series Office, 1972 (Chowkhamba Sanskrit Studies, vol. LXXXV).

Sharma P.V., *Introduction to dravyaguṇa (Indian Pharmacology)*, Varanasi, Chaukhamba Orientalia, 1976.

Sharma P.V., *Fruits and Vegetables in Ancient India*, Varanasi, Chaukhamba Orientalia, 1979.

Sharma S., *The System of Ayurveda*. Reprinted, Delhi, Neeraj Publishing House, 1983.

Sharma S., *Āyurvedic Medicine Past and Present*, edited by K. Sharma, Third edition, Varanasi, Krishnadas Academy, 1987.

Singhal G.D., Sharma Gaur D., *Surgical Ethics in Āyurveda*, Varanasi, Chaukhamba Sanskrit Series Office, 1963.

Srivastava G.P., *History of Indian Pharmacy*, with a foreword from Dr. George Urdang, Calcutta, Pindars Ltd., 1954.

Subba Reddy D.V., *Glimpses of Health and Medicine in Mauryan Empire*, Hyderabad, Osmania Medical College, 1966.

Udupa K.N., Chaturvedi G.N., Tripathi S.N., *Advances in Research in Indian Medicine*, Varanasi, Banaras Hindu University, 1970.

Vohora S.B., Research on Medicinal Plants in India : A Review of Reviews, *Curare*, 12, 1989, p. 16-22.

Wujastyk D., *The Roots of Āyurveda, Selections from Sanskrit Medical Writings*, New Delhi, Penguin Books India, 1998.

Zimmermann F., *Le discours des remèdes au pays des épices*, Paris, Editions Payot, 1989.

Zimmermann F., *The Jungle and the Aroma of Meats: An Ecological Theme in Hindu Medicine*, Delhi, Motilal Banarsidass, 1999 (Indian Medical Tradition, vol. 4).

Zysk K.G., *Medicine in the Veda, Religious healing in the Veda*, Delhi, Motilal Banarsidass, 1996 (Indian Medical Tradition, vol. 1).

Zysk K.G., *Asceticism and healing in ancient India: medicine in the Buddhist monastery*, Delhi, Motilal Banarsidass, 1998 (Indian Medical Tradition, vol. 2).